3D Histology Evaluation of Dermatologic Surgery

Helmut Breuninger • Patrick Adam

3D Histology
Evaluation
of Dermatologic Surgery

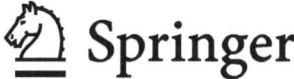

Springer

Helmut Breuninger
Universitätsklinikum Tübingen
Hautklinik
Tübingen
Germany

Patrick Adam
Universitätsklinikum Tübingen
Pathologie und Pathologische
Anatomie
Tübingen
Germany

ISBN 978-1-4471-4437-3   ISBN 978-1-4471-4438-0   (eBook)
DOI 10.1007/978-1-4471-4438-0
Springer London Heidelberg New York Dordrecht

Library of Congress Control Number: 2013938491

Printed on acid-free paper

Springer is part of Springer Science+Business Media (www.springer.com)

About the Authors

Helmut Breuninger, MD, is a specialist for surgery and dermatology as well and worked since 32 years as dermatosurgeon at the Department of Dermatology of the University of Tübingen. In this time, more than 50,000 malignant skin tumors have been treated in his Department of Dermatosurgery, which is specialized for 3D histological procedures, and a high number of respective international publications with very high case numbers have been published. Here the collaboration with the histopathology was crucial.

Patrick Adam, MD, is a specialist for pathology in the Department of Pathology working tight together with the Department of Dermatology and has more than 12 years of experience in histopathologic diagnosis of skin tumors. During this time, he has established schemes of sectioning for the histopathologic workup.

Acknowledgements

First of all, we thank Mr. Grant Weston, Senior Editor from Springer Medicine, London, who had the idea to this book and who supported the authors during the work on this book. Special thanks to Dr. Holger Breuninger of the University of Oxford for reading and editing this book.

We would like to thank the following colleagues who all had given a lot of very important suggestions (in alphabetic order): Franziska Eberle, MD; Hans-Martin Häfner, MD; Malte Hübner, MD; Matin Röcken, MD; Camillo Roldan, MD; Saskia Schnabl, MD; Ugur Uslu; and Daniel Wilder, MD.

Last but not least, we will thank the Springer publishing team for having done a superb job with the publication.

Contents

Chapter 1
Introduction

About This Book

In the past, a lot of individual surgery procedures and histo-pathological investigation for skin tumors have been extensively discussed in the literature, e.g., Mohs' surgery and methods of other disciplines as well. This interdisciplinary book attempts to summarize and compare the most commonly used methods in order to give the reader the most comprehensive and complete overview of the current state of the art in the field. To this end, the basic principles of various surgical methods and following histological workups of the complete 3D tumor margins will be described and extensively graphically illustrated to allow a better understanding. Furthermore, also more complex treatments of larger tumors will be discussed and comprehensively illustrated.

It should be noted that all methods described here are exchangeable and can be freely combined much to the liking of the executing surgeon and pathologist. Clinically, there are only minor differences between most of the described procedures in this book. This will allow the reader to come up with his or her own preferred choice of surgery and histological control which will help to assess and streamline the currently used workflow.

Not only surgical skills and histological preparations and evaluations are important for a successful and efficient treatment of various malignant skin tumors, also a good knowledge of local patterns of infiltration is required to achieve complete

H. Breuninger, P. Adam, *3D Histology Evaluation of Dermatologic Surgery*, DOI 10.1007/978-1-4471-4438-0_1, © Springer-Verlag London 2013

excision. All tumors may show an irregular, often asymmetric, mainly horizontal subclinical infiltration with a lateral extent of zero to several centimeters within the epidermis, dermis, and upper subcutaneous tissue. When in-depth infiltrations are present, they are often asymmetric as well and hard to determine before excision. Up to now, these tumor outgrowths are only detectable by a histological evaluation. 3D histology is highly sensitive and can detect even very small tumor infiltrations; therefore, very narrow margins can be taken for excision. This helps sparing healthy skin as only a subsequently targeted re-excision will be necessary to remove all of the asymmetric tumor infiltrations. Therefore, the resulting defect will be as small as possible and as large as necessary. The resulting shape of the defect can be adapted to the requirement of the rules for aesthetic surgical defect closure.

Also the organization of the workflow, the scheme of documentation used, and the available infrastructure greatly influence the efficiency and accuracy of the procedure. This directly improves the patient's welfare, as less and more targeted surgical procedures with a high reproducibility can be performed. Hence, the importance of workflow organization and documentation cannot be underestimated. Consequently, an entire chapter of this book is dedicated to this critical aspect of skin tumor treatment.

The main emphasis of this book lays on a thorough and comprehensive illustration of the methods. Therefore, the illustrations should be self-explaining and may not require any further explanations. However, every figure is accompanied by comprehensive description in order to give the reader the best and most complete introduction to all discussed methods.

What Is 3D Histology?

3D histology provides a complete 3D representation of the margins of a tumor specimen on histological slides (Table 1.1). This eliminates diagnostic gaps and provides maximum sensitivity in identifying tumor outgrowths. The method is used to

TABLE 1.1 Definition of 3D histology

1. Complete 3D margins of a tumor specimen in histological slides

2. No diagnostic gaps

3. The highest sensitivity to make tumor outgrowths topographical visible

4. Tumor-positive areas are removed by step-by-step re-excisions until the margins are clear

5. Saving healthy tissue. Minimal invasive surgery

confirm tumor-free margins or, in case of an incomplete tumor resection, to make even very small infiltrated areas visible with topographic orientation (Fig. 1.1).

It should be mentioned that in the figures of this book, tumor outgrowths which might have been missed in the first excision are highlighted as brown spots at the margins of the tumor specimens and in the resulting defect for better visualization of the reader. These outgrowths are clinically invisible and can only be seen histologically *after* staining with H&E. They are intended to show the complexities and variability of tumor outgrowths and should help to understand the importance of 3D histology.

The basic principle of 3D histology is the conversion from the 3D structure of the tumor-specimen margins into a 2D view of histological sections to detect tumor infiltrations. The 3D margins are flattened with their outside down and then cut into pieces, suitable for histopathological procedures of cryo- or paraffin sections (see Chaps. 2 and 3). Only tumors with a continuous infiltration pattern are suitable for this method, but not those with a discontinuous spread (see Chap. 7).

Tumor-infiltrated areas can then be removed step by step by targeted re-excisions until the margins are clear, thus sparing healthy tissue. This minimal invasive surgery ensures that the defect will be as small as possible especially in difficult localizations. The next figure gives an overview over the workflow using 3D histology and the corresponding chapters of this book in which extensive explanations will be given (Fig. 1.2).

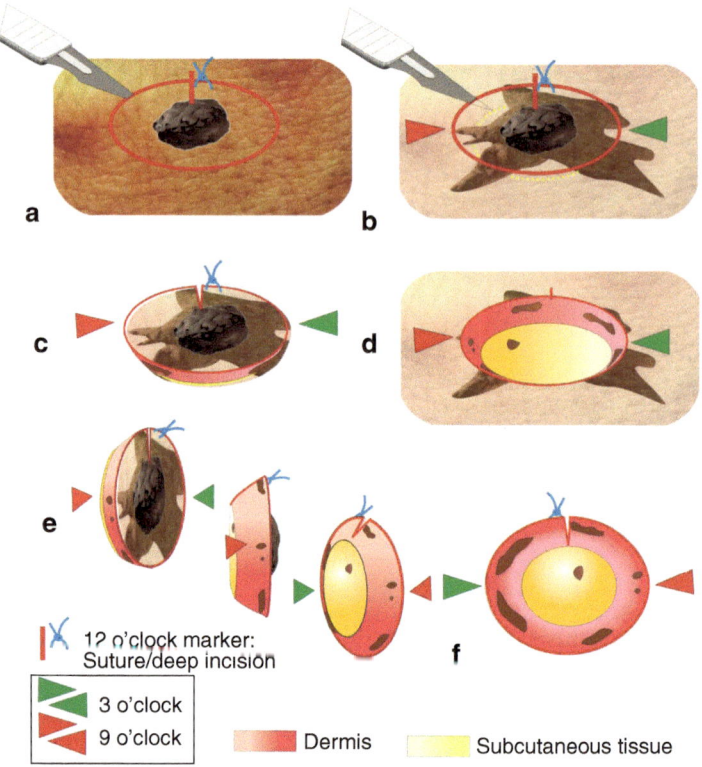

FIGURE 1.1 Tumor with subclinical infiltrations. After excision and flipping over, the 3D margin outside of the specimen can be seen. (**a**) The clinically visible tumor with excisional margins. A suture or deep incision at 12 o'clock relative to the patient's top of the head serves as a landmark. Tumor resection line in *red*. (**b**) Subclinically, normally invisible tumor infiltrations are shown in *brown* for purposes of illustration. (**c**) The excised tumor with its surrounding tissue and 3D borders. (**d**) The defect after excision. (**e**) Illustration of the "bowl-shaped" tumor specimen as it is flipped over to see its reverse side. *Colored arrowheads* serve for orientation (*green arrowheads* 3 o'clock, *red arrows* 9 o'clock). (**f**) The complete 3D view of the excisional margins from beneath with subclinical, infiltration sites in *brown*. These infiltrations only become visible after histological staining

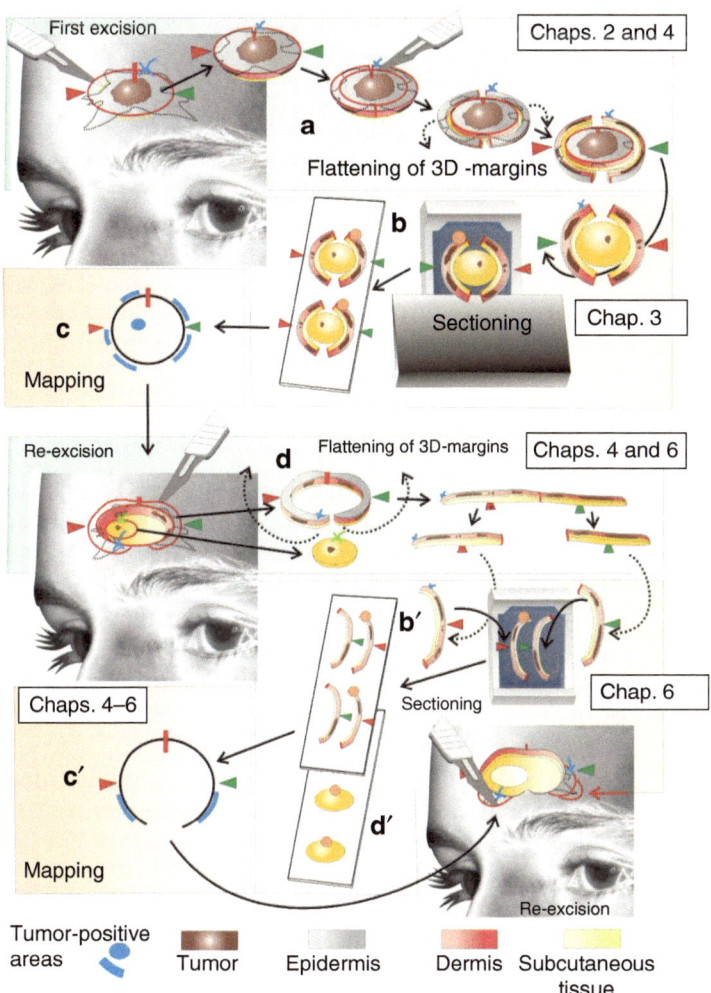

FIGURE 1.2 Short workflow of using 3D histology. Tumor excision, flattening of the 3D margins, sectioning, mapping, and re-excisions. (**a**) Excision of the tumor of Fig. 1.1 and flattening of its 3D margin to a 2D plane using incisions (see Chaps. 2 and 4). (**b** and **b′**) Embedding and sectioning and resulting histological slides (see Chap. 3). (**c** and **c′**) Mapping of tumor-positive areas: margins 1–5, 7–12 o'clock, and base central toward 9 o'clock (see Chaps. 5, 6, and 7). (**d**) First re-excision and flattening of the margin and base with their outside down (see Chaps. 4 and 6) and (**d′**) second and third re-excision

Thus, the aim of the 3D histology to detect all outgrowths of a tumor should be standard for every surgical procedure. The selection of the techniques used in 3D histology, however, strongly depends on the expertise and personal preferences of the local cooperating surgeon and pathologist. Both have to be specially trained, and a standardized workflow should be established individually in each department. It is crucial to define responsibilities for each person or department involved. Otherwise, communication errors, resulting in missing of tumor outgrowths, may severely endanger the patients' health.

A Few Historical Details

3D tumor histology was introduced in 1941 in the USA by the surgeon F. Mohs, initially in the form of chemosurgery for basal cell carcinomas. Mohs first used a fixative zinc chloride paste prior to performing the actual excision [1]. Up to this time, it has been standard totally to excise a malignant tumor with wide margins whenever possible in one step completely. Mohs was the first to cut out a malignant tumor in steps. His concept of stepwise surgical excision has proven to be very safe. In 1974, Tromovitch introduced a technique in which the excision was performed under local anesthesia, and histological analysis was done by cryo-sectioning using cryostat [2]. Mohs called this procedure "microscopically controlled surgery (MCS)" until 1985 [3, 4].

Later, the term "MCS" was also used for different techniques using serial horizontal or vertical cuts of the tumor specimen with a topographic orientation. Sequential vertical cuts every 1–3 mm are done. Representative sections are then taken from these tissue slices. Thin sections can allow so far sufficient sensitivity, but diagnostic gaps must be wider; the broader the cuts are spaced, the greater the tumor specimen will be.

To differentiate methods with complete histological evaluation from those with gaps, D. Jones in 1974 coined the term "micrographic surgery" [5]. In 1985, the American Society of Mohs' micrographic surgery was founded to distinguish

TABLE 1.2 Various methods of incision

1. Chemosurgery by Mohs [1]

2. Systematic histological control of the tumor bed in paraffin procedure [6]

3. Fresh tissue technique [2]

4. Histographic surgery with horizontal serial sections [7]

5. Histologic control of excised tissue edges [8, 13]

6. Square technique: geometrical excision of tumor and margin [14]

7. Perimeter technique: first excision of a margin strip, leaving the tumor in situ [15]

8. Muffin technique: excision of the tumor with margins, perpendicular incision of margin strips, and flattening in one piece with the base [16]

Mohs' method from other methods of complete histological margin control the earliest from 1963 [6–8]. Later, colleagues of Mohs created the term "Mohs' surgery" [9–11], which is slightly misleading as the procedure is not a special type of surgery but rather a method for histologically evaluating the borders of a tumor specimen in 3D and performing stepwise surgical excisions until clear margins are proven. Using automated staining, the surgeon basically functions as his or her own pathologist, can assess the sections within an hour, and can immediately perform any necessary re-excision. However, this personal union is not available in many countries. For more information on this issue, the new book about Mohs' micrographic surgery is recommended [12].

Various alternatives for histological examination of excised tissue margins are described in the literature [6–8, 13–16] (Table 1.2). In contrast to the here described Mohs' micrographic surgery, however, these techniques are performed with vertical incisions. This kind of excision shows a vertical cut of epidermis, dermis, and subcutaneous layer. Therefore, it is adapted to the pattern of horizontal spread of most of the malignant skin tumors and advantageous for the defect closure with sutures. In addition, these procedures differ in the way the 3D margins of a tumor specimen are flattened to convert them into a 2D plane to ensure R0 resection (histologically proved complete excision) by histological sections of the complete margins. The complete 3D incision margins of a tumor specimen become visible in stained histological sections [17]. Thus, the term three-dimensional histology (3D histology) was created in the literature [18]. The usefulness of the chosen technique depends on the expertise and experience of the surgeon and his pathologist and their familiarity with the respective method.

To avoid confusion and misunderstandings, all of these procedures must be documented using special locally adapted protocols (clear rules of embedding and/or drawings) in order to allow topographic depiction of tumor-positive areas in the margins. All use a topographic marker to precisely localize tumor-positive parts at the margin. The results can be documented in the form using clock times (measured from a marker at 12 o'clock in relation to the body axis) or topographical drawings.

Why Do We Need 3D Histology?

Complete removal of a locally growing tumor is the only way to ensure a cure. Up to now, even with modern techniques (ultrasound, confocal laser microscopy, fluorescence photo diagnostic), it remains difficult if not impossible to determine the precise borders of a skin tumor pre- as well as intraoperatively. On the other hand, in most cases, tumors show an asymmetric pattern of infiltration, often consisting of very fine tumor strands. Therefore, it is necessary to evaluate the entire periphery of the excised tumor specimen.

Such gap-free methods have the highest capacity to ensure R0 resection as these detect even very small tumor infiltrations. Therefore, very small margin widths can be taken for excision allowing to spare healthy skin by taking the asymmetric areas of tumor infiltration into account. This minimal invasive technique also results in better defect closure with good aesthetic results [19] and a higher cure rate compared to other tumor treatments [20].

References

1. Mohs FE. Chemosurgery: a microscopically controlled method of cancer excision. Arch Surg. 1941;42:279–81.
2. Tromovitch TA, Stegmann SJ. Microscopically controlled excision of skin tumours. Arch Dermatol. 1974;110:231–2.
3. Mohs FE. Chemosurgery: a microscopically controlled surgery. Springfield: Charles C. Thomas; 1978. p. 249–50.
4. Mohs FE, Snow SN. Microscopically controlled surgery for suqamous cell carcinoma of the lip. Surg Gynecol Obstet. 1985;160:37–41.
5. Brodland DG, Amonette R, Hanke WC, Robbins P. The history of Mohs micrographic surgery. Dermatol Surg. 2000;26:303–7.
6. Drepper H. Systematic histological control of the tumor-bed as an advance in the operative removal of deep facial skin cancers. Hautarzt. 1963;14:420–3.
7. Burg G, Hirsch R, Konz B, Braun-Falco O. Histographic surgery. Accuracy of visual assessment of the margins of basal-cell epithelioma. J Dermatol Surg Oncol. 1975;1:21–5.
8. Breuninger H. Histologic control of excised tissue edges in the operative treatment of basal-cell carcinomas. J Dermatol Surg Oncol. 1984;10:724–8.
9. Miller PK, Roenigk RK, Brodland DG, Randle HW. Cutaneous micrographic surgery: Mohs procedure. Mayo Clin Proc. 1992;67:971–80.
10. Dinehart SM, Dodge R, Stanley WE, Franks HH, Pollack SV. Basal cell carcinoma treated with Mohs surgery. J Dermatol Surg Oncol. 1992;18:560–6.
11. Shriner DL, McCoy DK, Golberg DJ, Wagner RF. Mohs micrographic surgery. J Am Acad Dermatol. 1998;39:79–97.
12. Keyvan N, editor. Mohs micrographic surgery. London: Springer; 2012.
13. Breuninger H, Schaumburg-Lever G. Control of excisional margins by conventional histopathological techniques in the treatment of skin tumours. An alternative to Mohs' technique. J Pathol. 1988;154:167–71.
14. Johnson TM, Headington JT, Baker SR, Lowe L. Usefulness of staged excision for lentigo maligna and lentigo maligna melanoma: the square procedure. J Am Acad Dermatol. 1997;37:758–64.
15. Mahoney MH, Joseph M, Temple CL. The perimeter technique for lentigo maligna: an alternative to Mohs micrographic surgery. J Surg Oncol. 2005;1:120–5.

16. Möhrle M, Breuninger H. The Muffin technique – an alternative to Mohs' micrographic surgery. J Dtsch Dermatol Ges. 2006;4:1080–4.
17. Leibovitch I, Huilgol SC, Selva D, Hill D, Richards S, Paver R. Basalcellcarcinoma treated with Mohs micrographic surgery in Australia: II. Experience over 10 years. J Am Acad Dermatol. 2005; 53:452–7.
18. Moehrle M, Breuninger H, Röcken M. A confusing world: what to call histology of three-dimensional tumour margins? J Eur Acad Dermatol Venereol. 2007;21:591–5.
19. Eberle FC, Schippert W, Trilling B, Röcken M, Breuninger H. Cosmetic results of histoFigureally excision of non-melanoma skin cancer in the head and neck region. J Dtsch Dermatol Ges. 2005;3:109–12.
20. Häfner HM, Breuninger H, Moehrle M, Trilling B, Krimmel M. 3D histology-guided surgery for basal cell carcinoma and squamous cell carcinoma: recurrence rates and clinical outcome. Int J Oral Maxillofac Surg. 2011;40:943–8.

Chapter 2
The Basics for Excision and Flattening

In this chapter, the basic principles of tumor excisions will be discussed. By introducing several different methods for tumor excisions and converting 3D margins to a 2D plane, the reader will be given the opportunity to develop her/his own preferred procedure. It should be noted that the choice of method is mainly influenced by the preferences of the executing surgeon, the interaction between surgical team and pathology, and the histological procedure chosen which will be discussed later in this book (Chap. 5).

Skin tumors can be excised by using either an oblique or vertical incision. Both of these methods will be introduced using examples of small tumor samples only for better understanding. It is relatively easy to scale the methods introduced here up to larger tumor sizes. To this end, it is simply necessary to divide the tumor excisions into smaller pieces so that they will be the right size for the histological embedding procedures which follow (see Chap. 4).

Excising the Tumor and Conversion of 3D Margins to a 2D Plane

In this section, various techniques for excising tumors and the following conversion of the 3D margins to a plane by flattening them down will be discussed in detail. For a better understanding, all procedures are also illustrated in either 3D

H. Breuninger, P. Adam, *3D Histology Evaluation* 11
of Dermatologic Surgery, DOI 10.1007/978-1-4471-4438-0_2,
© Springer-Verlag London 2013

or 2D graphics. The excision of the tumor is followed by the conversion of the 3D margins of the sample into a 2D specimen, which can be used for histological diagnostics (3D histology). It is crucial for orientation to set a marker at the excised tissue. A suture or deep incision at 12 o'clock relative to the patient's top of the head serves as a landmark. An incision is sufficient if the surgeon performs the division, flattening, and embedding of the tissue; a suture is necessary if the pathologist does this (see Chap. 5).

Oblique Excision of the Tumor

Excising the tumor with an angled section greatly enhances this flattening of the 3D margins to a 2D tissue plane, and this is why Mohs' method uses this approach. Once all margins are cleared of the tumor, Mohs' surgeons prefer a secondary wound healing. Hereby, the oblique margins facilitate this secondary wound healing and lead in a great deal of smaller defects to well-acceptable aesthetic results.

Two-Step Oblique Excision and Flattening of the 3D Margins to a Plane

In a first step, the tumor is clinically completely removed for diagnosis by curettage (Fig. 2.1a). To remove the subclinical outgrowths as well, the surrounding tissue is excised in a second step. To mark the orientation of the excised specimen, it is important to set one or more markers prior to excision (one at least at 12 o'clock in relation to the body axis relative to the top of the patient's head). Then, the tumor "shell," i.e., the margin, is excised with a circular oblique 45° incision (Fig. 2.1b). Here the scalpel is angled away from the tumor so that the circular excision removes a tissue bowl-shaped cone and will leave a complementary bowl-shaped defect on the patient.

The 3D bowl-shaped tumor specimen of the excision (magnified for better visualization in Fig. 2.1b′) can be easily converted into a 2D plane. By cutting the "bowl" of tissue in, e.g., crosswise 90° angles (Fig. 2.1c), the sample can be pressed

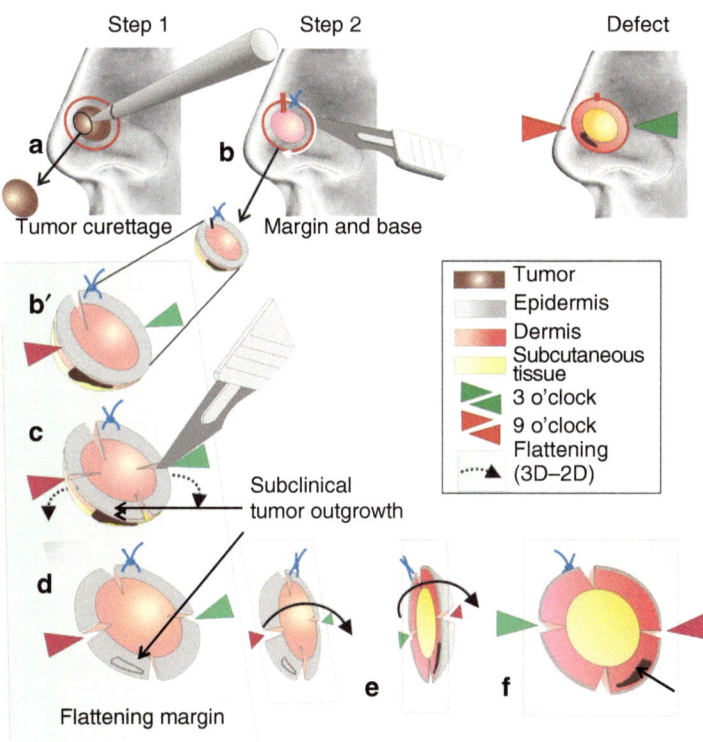

FIGURE 2.1 Two-step oblique excision and flattening of 3D margins to a 2D plane. When flipped over, the 2D excisional margins are seen

flat to level the slanted margins with the base (Fig. 2.1c bended arrows). In doing so, the excised material is converted into a 2D sample with the entire outside of the specimen facing down in one plane as it is required for sectioning (Fig. 2.1d). In this example, a tumor outgrowth is shown for illustration only. This tissue is macroscopically invisible and therefore indistinguishable from other tissue. However, it will become visible after staining in a histological section. To show the reader the flat underside of the tumor for better imagination, i.e., the outside of the tissue "bowl," the specimen is flipped over (Fig. 2.1e, f) (in Chap. 3, Fig. 3.8, this will be the view at the microtome). Note that landmarks for orientation at 3 o'clock and 9 o'clock are now reversed, and the tumor outgrowth is mirrored (Fig. 2.3f). Now, embedding, horizontal slicing, and staining can be performed, and after staining, tumor-positive areas can be detected. Re-resections can be carried out very precisely.

Two-Dimensional Scheme of Oblique Excision and Flattening 3D Margins

For better visualization of the conversion from 3D tissue into a 2D plane, the movement is illustrated here in a 2D scheme. First, the tumor is removed for diagnosis by curettage (Fig. 2.2a). This step is followed by the 45° oblique circular excision of the tumor "shell," i.e., margin (Fig. 2.2b). Due to the oblique cutting parts of the tumor, outgrowths may be missed and remain on the right side of the defect. The resulting bowl-shaped piece of tissue can be easily flattened by a few cuts, e.g., 90° steps (Fig. 2.2c).

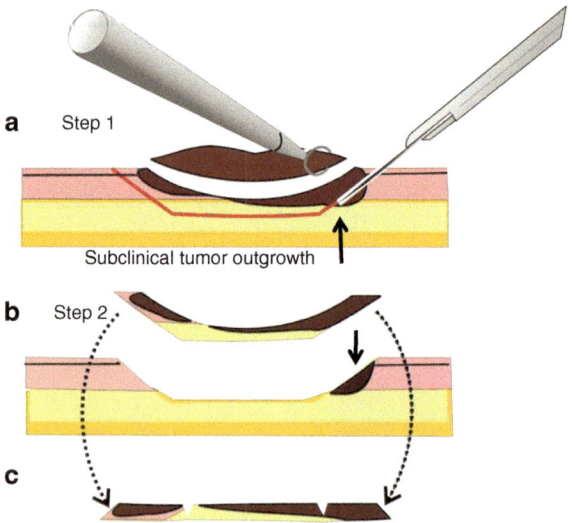

a   Step 1

Subclinical tumor outgrowth

b   Step 2

c

FIGURE 2.2 Two-dimensional scheme of oblique excision and flattening of 3D margins to a plane

Vertical Excision of the Tumor

A vertical, 90° incision is very commonly used by surgeons. It is adapted to the pattern of horizontal spread of most of the malignant skin tumors within the dermis and upper subcutaneous tissue and does not compromise the adaption of the wound edges by sutures. To convert the 90° margin of vertical incisions into a plane, few modifications in the preparation of the excised tissue have to be accommodated.

Two-Step Vertical Excision and Flattening of the 3D Margins to a Plane

The first step should be the removal of the central tumor tissue for diagnostics. The tumor is removed with an incision leaving a 2–3 mm margin to the planned outline of the excision. Then the tumor center is cut out, either by sissors or a scalpel, leving deeper layers in the patient (Fig. 2.3a). Figure 2.3b shows the resulting flat defect. A marker is set at 12 o'clock.

In a second step, the surrounding tumor margins of 2–3 mm in width can be excised with a vertical incision together with the deeper, central tissue parts which can be removed using either scissors or a scalpel. This resulting "cake tin"-shaped margin sample (Fig. 2.3b, b′) with a vertical edge is not as easily converted into a flat sample as the "bowl"-shaped samples. To facilitate the conversion in this case, the vertical edges of the margin sample should be cut with 90° at the 12 and 6 o'clock positions deeply with all layers to allow stretching of the margin strip (Fig. 2.3c). With some additional crosswise incisions at various positions (Fig. 2.3d), it would be possible to flatten the edges and bring them into the same plane as the central tissue with the epidermis pointing outwards (Fig. 2.2e). In this way, the outside of the margin will be facing down as it is required for sectioning. To show the reader this flat underside of the specimen, it is flipped over (Fig. 2.3e, f) (during this step of the procedure, this flipping is not necessary). Note that landmarks for orientation at 3 o'clock and 9 o'clock are now reversed, and the

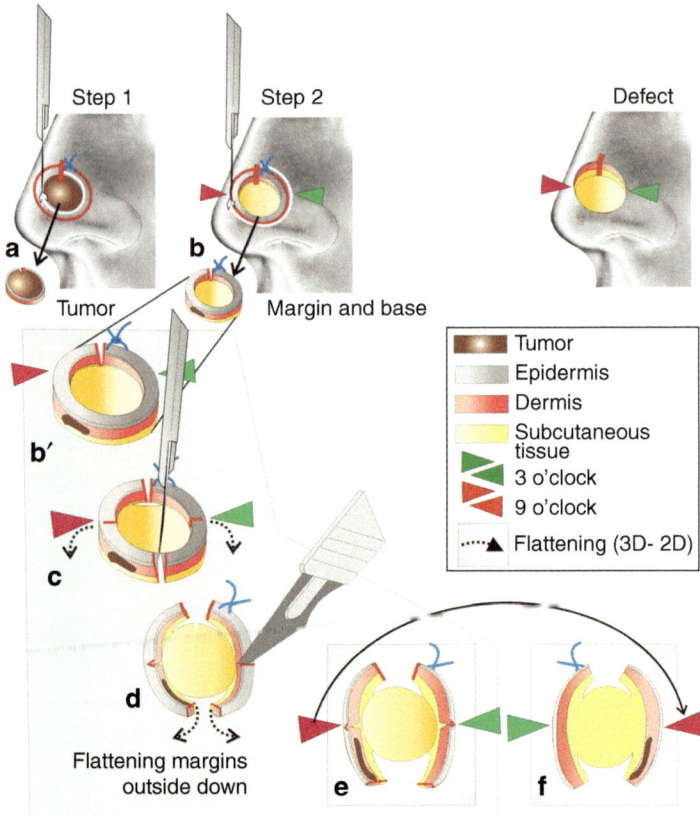

FIGURE 2.3 Two-step vertical excision and flattening of 3D margin strips to a 2D plane. When flipped over, the 2D excisional margins are seen

tumor outgrowth is mirrored (Fig. 2.3f). Now, embedding, horizontal slicing, and staining can be performed making tumor-positive areas detectable. Re-operations can be carried out topographically targeted. The resulting deeper defect with vertical edges is to be closed with common methods of plastic surgery.

This flattening should be done carefully, and compared with the oblique excised samples, it needs slightly more practice. If the sample is insufficient in a plane, epidermal tissue might be lost in the histological sections making a full histological workup more difficult. Cutting off the margin rim completely facilitates flattening (Figs. 2.5 and 2.7).

It is worth mentioning that besides the differences in the procedure, also differences in the tumor diagnostics can be found. The slightly minor quality of the curettage used for diagnostics in the oblique excision can cause difficulties whereas the entire middle part of the tumor of the vertical section allows for a more complete picture of the tumor growth. In some instances like the squamous cell carcinoma, the measurement of the tumor thickness, which cannot be determined in curettages, influences the prognosis (Brantsch).

Two-Dimensional Scheme of Vertical Excision and Flattening 3D Margins

For better visualization of the conversion of vertical excisions from 3D to 2D, the entire procedure is shown here in a 2D scheme. First, the tumor is excised as described in Fig. 2.3 for tumor diagnostics (Fig. 2.4a). Then a strip of the safety margin 2–3 mm wide and the deeper tissue beneath the excised tumor part by a vertical and horizontal is cut (Fig. 2.4a). The vertical margin is bent down with incisions as described in Fig. 2.3 into a flat surface (Fig. 2.4b, c). After this procedure, the margins and the bottom (with outer side down) are now in a one plane and ready for histological sectioning (Fig. 2.4c).

Using the basic vertical incision, several minor variations of excisions have been developed over the time. In the following, some of the most common variations for vertical excisions will be described.

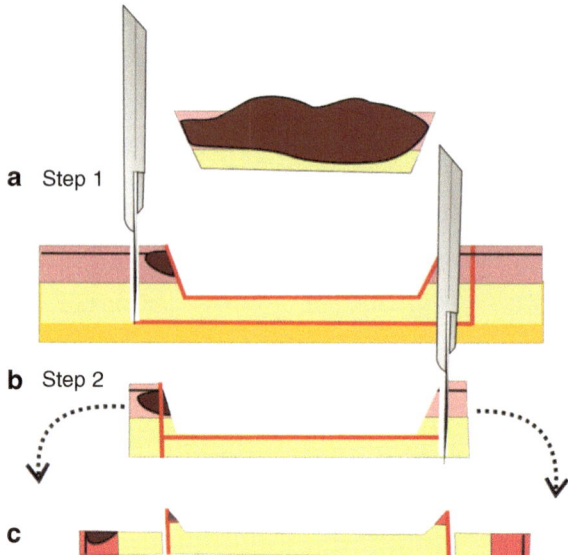

FIGURE 2.4 Two-dimensional scheme of vertical excision and flattening of 3D margins to a plane

Three-Step Vertical Excision and Flattening of the 3D Margins

Rather than removing the tumor margins in one step, some surgeons prefer to remove the central tumor, the surrounding margins, and the base in three independent excisions. As always, a marker is set at 12 o' clock (incision or suture marker, here in blue). In this example, an additional suture marker (violet) at the patient's site of the defect is set to facilitate later orientation. Then first, the central tumor is removed as described before leaving back the margins and the base (Fig. 2.5a). Next, the tumor margins are excised in two steps. First, a strip of the margin of about 2–3 mm is cut vertically from the border. The blue suture marker identifies

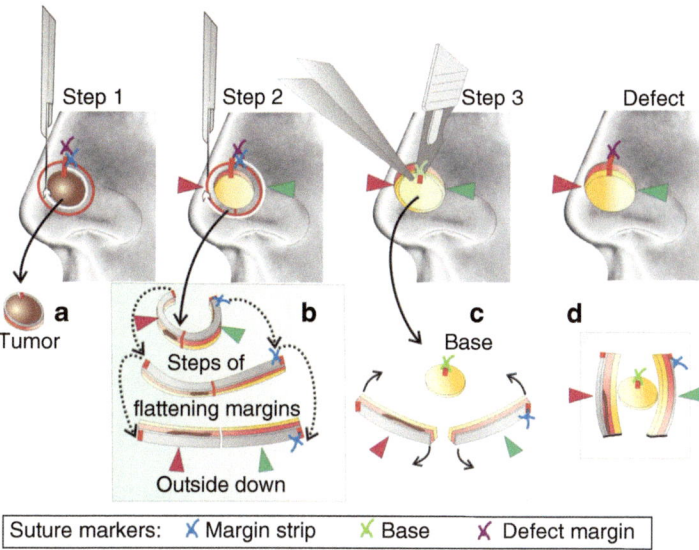

FIGURE 2.5 Three-step vertical excision and flattening of margin strips and base to a plane. Additional 12 o'clock marker at the patient

the beginning in 1 o'clock direction. The strip is pressed flat with its outside down for histological processing (Fig. 2.5b). Then the suture-marked base (green) of the tumor is excised using surgical forceps and scissors or a scalpel (Fig. 2.5c). As this procedure separates the base and the side margins of the tumor, the isolated excisional margins can easily be brought into one plane (Fig. 2.5c). Dividing the side margins into two pieces and placing them next to the tumor base with the epidermis pointing outward is enough to obtain a full view of the margins in one histological section (Fig. 2.5d). However, as this procedure is performed in three independent excisions, there is also three times bleeding to be expected.

Please note different colors of the suture markers are not necessary in reality.

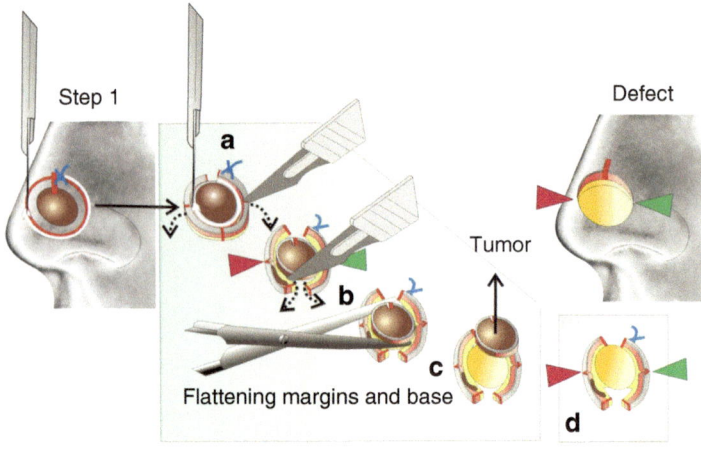

FIGURE 2.6 One-step vertical excision and flattening margins to a plane. Removal of tumor center leaving base in place (muffin technique)

One-Step Vertical Excision and Flattening of the 3D Margins (Muffin Technique)

To avoid multiple bleedings and multiple excisions, the central tumor, the safety margins, and the base can also be excised in one step. A 12 o'clock marker is placed first. Now the tumor is excised with a vertical incision together with the planned safety margin and the base (Fig. 2.6a). To separate the vertical margins of the excised specimen, an incision is placed around the margin creating a rim of 2–3 mm. Within this cutoff margin sample, crosswise 90° incisions are placed as described in Fig. 2.3 (Fig. 2.6a, b) to allow stretching the margin strip with its outside down and flatten it with the epidermis pointing out. It looks like removing the paper sleeve of a muffin (muffin technique). Now the central tumor can be removed leaving the tumor base intact using scissors or a scalpel and submitted to diagnostics (Fig. 2.6c). In this way, the excisional margins and the base are one connected flatted specimen for histological sectioning (Fig. 2.6d). The resulting sections represent the entire outside of the tumor in one section. Hence,

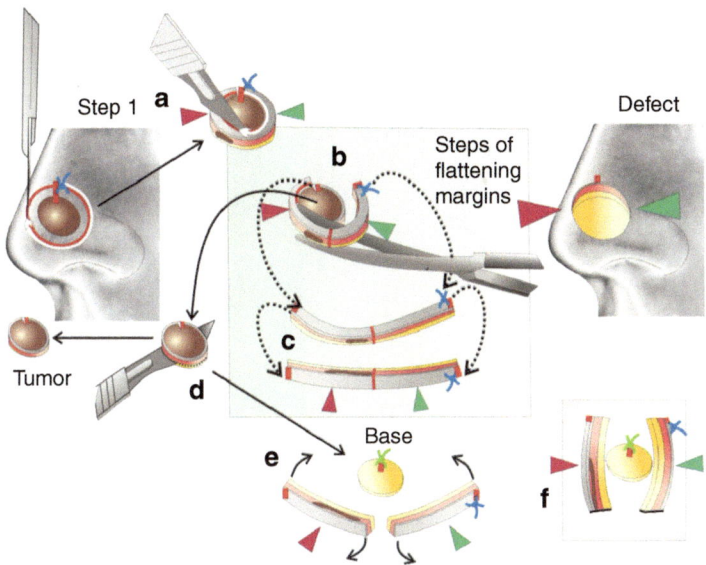

FIGURE 2.7 One-step vertical excision, cutting lateral margins strips and base to a plane (strip technique)

orientation relative to the patient will be easier, and less effort in processing several samples will be required.

A disadvantage of this method is that the flattening of the 90° margins relative to the base might need some practice.

One-Step Vertical Excision, Cutting Lateral Strips and Base for Flattening (Strip Technique)

To circumvent the potential difficulties in flattening, the safety margins and base can be prepared separately from an excised tumor specimen. First the tumor, with a marker set at 12 o'clock position, is excised together with the subcutaneous tissue and a safety margin by a vertical cut (Fig. 2.7a). To separate the margin and central tumor from such specimens, the 2–3 mm wide margin strips can be removed using a scalpel and or scissors (Fig. 2.7a, b) so that the entire margin of

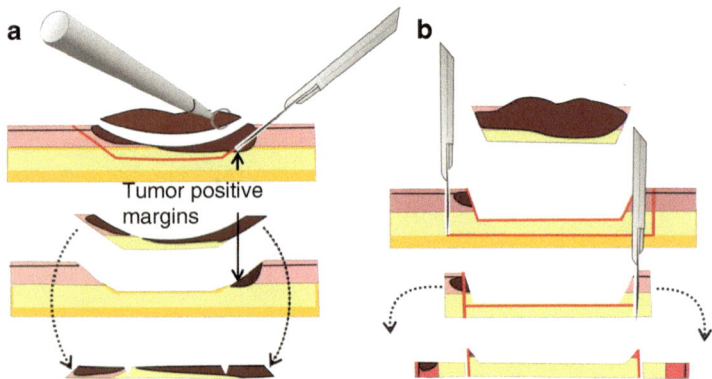

FIGURE 2.8 Two-dimensional schemes, comparing oblique (**a**) and vertical (**b**) incision and flattening of 3D margins

the specimen is represented in one strip starting left from the 12 o'clock suture marker (Fig. 2.7b, c). This strip can then be laid flat with the outside of the surface facing down (Fig. 2.7c). Following the removal of the margins, the tumor center with its base was left behind (Fig. 2.7d). From this specimen, the bottom is cut away (Fig. 2.7d, e) and the tissue left above can be taken for tumor diagnostics. The bottom (base) and the entire margin of the excised sample are now transformed from its 3D outside into a 2D specimen with the outside facing down (Fig. 2.7e). Now, embedding, horizontal slicing, and staining can be performed, and after staining, tumor-positive areas can be detected (Fig. 2.7f).

Two-Dimensional Scheme, Comparing Oblique and Vertical Incisions and Flattening of 3D Margins

Here the differences between the two above described methods of incision are compared in a 2D scheme side by side. On the left (Fig. 2.8a), the oblique excision procedure is shown. The excision at a 45° angle may compromise defect closure techniques and result in more frequent tumor-positive findings. On the right, the vertical excision procedure is shown (Fig. 2.8b).

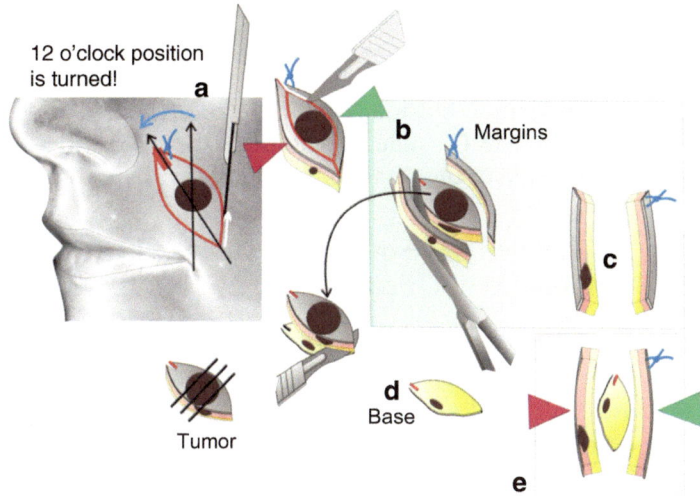

FIGURE 2.9 Spindle-shaped vertical excision and flattening of the margins. 12 o'clock marker at the upper point

These basic principles, oblique and vertical excision, tumor and safety margin excision in multiple excisions, or one with following preparation of the central tumor, are the core of any surgical procedure for skin tumors. In the following, two other variants of excision methods using vertical excisions are described.

Vertical Excision of a Spindle-Shaped Tumor Specimen

In some cases, depending on the location and size of the tumor, it might be advantageous to do the excision of the tumor in a vertical spindle rather than a round-shaped cut. The procedure here is very comparable to the round-shaped excision. As before, the tumor is excised with a safety margin together with the subcutaneous tissue with two spindle-shaped incisions around the tumor. In this instance, the marker should be positioned at the top of the spindle and may therefore deviate from the 12 o'clock position which has to be documented (see arrows in Fig. 2.9a). To separate the side margins, two 2–3 mm wide strips are cut from the borders with a scalpel and or a scissors (Fig. 2.9b, c). The bottom of the excised tumor specimen is cut away as well (Fig. 2.9d). Now, the strips and bottom are placed with their outside down in a plane (Fig. 2.9e). Using this procedure, H&E stained sections can be taken from the complete outside of the tumor specimen.

Vertical Excision and Square Procedure, Two Possibilities of Orientation

To facilitate the flattening of the tumor margins, some surgeons prefer the removal of the tumor in a square-shaped specimen. Here the tumor with a safety margin is excised by four cuts forming a square. The 12 o'clock orientation differs in the examples shown (Fig. 2.10a, a'). The size of the square is determined by the largest visible outgrowth and the added

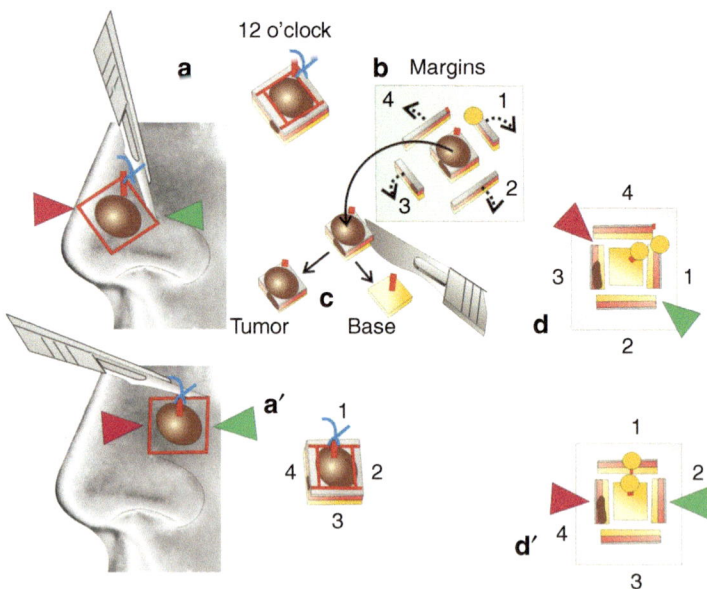

FIGURE 2.10 Vertical excision and square procedure, two possibilities of orientation cutting margins and base in a clockwise order

safety margin. From this square-shaped tumor specimen, the margins can now be easily cut away in a clockwise order (Fig. 2.10b). In the following, the bottom of the remaining specimen is separated and the tumor is sent for diagnostics (Fig. 2.10c). Now, embedding, horizontal slicing, and staining can begin, and after staining, tumor-positive areas can be detected (Fig. 2.10d, d'). Compared to spindle-shaped or round excisions, this method will result in straight margins which do not have to be bent down to be flat. Therefore, it will be slightly easier to recover sections representing the full margin. However, the major drawback to this method is the additional removal of potential healthy tissue. Also, the resulting square-shaped defect might be more difficult to close in some localizations. But on the other hand, the defect is ideal for closure by rhomboid flaps.

After the tumor is excised, the specimen is to be embedded and prepared for histological sectioning which will be discussed in the next chapter.

Chapter 3
Embedding and Sectioning

Following the excision of the tumor tissue and the conversion of the 3D tumor margins into a 2D plane, the tissue samples will have to be embedded and sectioned. There are two alternative commonly used techniques to prepare sections from the tumor samples which both produce sections suitable for a full diagnostics: paraffin sections or cryo-sections. In the following, both techniques will be discussed, and all required procedures for the preparation and the sectioning using either of them will be described and illustrated.

Paraffin- or Cryo-sections?

The main difference between the two methods is the time required to obtain results. However, there are considerable differences in quality as well. Depending on the sample size and other circumstances, each procedure has its own advantages and disadvantages (Table 3.1). With cryo-sections, the results may be available after only 20 min, but the procedure lasts considerably longer if tumor specimens are larger and more sections are necessary. Paraffin sections, on the other hand, require rapid tissue fixation in a 60 °C formalin solution for 2 h and then are only available after at least 20 h. This does not compromise the patient too much because skin excisions can be managed with local or tumescence local anesthesia and the defect can be easily bandaged. Therefore, a second

H. Breuninger, P. Adam, *3D Histology Evaluation*
of Dermatologic Surgery, DOI 10.1007/978-1-4471-4438-0_3,
© Springer-Verlag London 2013

TABLE 3.1 Cryo- versus paraffin sections

	Frozen sections	**Paraffin sections**
Advantages	Short waiting time	Routine procedure
	Inferior quality of stained specimens (more artifacts)	Very good quality of stained specimens
		Large surfaces of tissue can be worked on, up to 7.5 cm^2 or 25 mm in length
Disadvantages	Special equipment and experience	Longer waiting time
	Restricted surfaces, up to 5.3 cm^2 or 22 mm in length	
	High effort for large tumors	

excision step at another day or even later is easy to manage if the patient is hospitalized or lives in the surroundings.

The final choice between cryo- and paraffin sectioning used in the 3D histology depends on the expertise and special training of the surgeon and his collaboration with a pathologist. It is also influenced by the quality of the respective health-care system and the costs involved in each case.

As already described, for both procedures, the requirement is that the 3D outer surface of the tumor specimen is converted into a 2D plane sample to allow sectioning. Depending on the embedding technique, different embedding molds are commercially available which determine the sample size. Therefore, size of the plane of tissue varies between 7.5 cm^2 for paraffin technique and 5.3 cm^2 for the cryo-technique (Fig. 3.1).

Comparison of Embedding Cassettes

Commercially available standardized molds are used in all examples. On the left is the described cassette and mold for paraffin procedure (Fig. 3.1a) and on the right for comparison a standard plastic mold in the same magnification for single

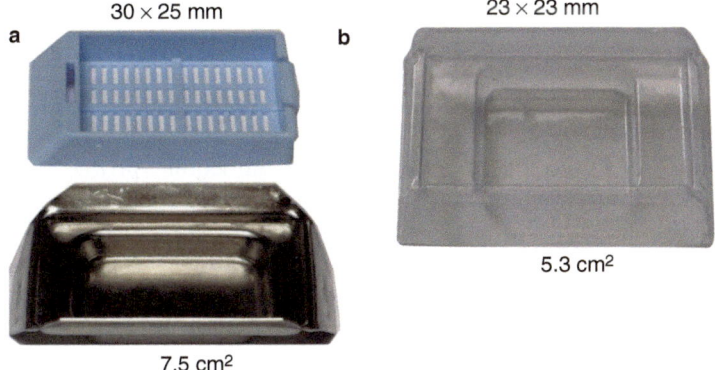

30 × 25 mm

23 × 23 mm

a

b

5.3 cm²

7.5 cm²

FIGURE 3.1 Comparison of embedding cassettes for paraffin technique (**a**) and cryo-technique (**b**)

use which can be used for cryo-technique (Fig. 3.1b). The size of the plane of tissue varies between 7.5 cm² for paraffin technique and 5.3 cm² for the cryo-technique.

The latter procedure may require several consecutive sectioning procedures to cover larger samples. In turn, this means that higher the effort, the larger the tumor sample is. Furthermore, frozen skin is difficult to cut, and a large specimen will have a lot of histological artifacts. Paraffin sections, on the other hand, can be processed up to 7.5 cm² in a very good quality taking the whole plane of the wax block. This means that the loss in time is compensated by the requirement of fewer sections, being of higher quality.

In the following, both methods will be discussed in detail. As before, all important procedures and steps are illustrated to help the reader.

Paraffin Sectioning

In this section, the preparation and sectioning of the tissue using paraffin embedding will be described. For paraffin sectioning, a prior formalin fixation of the samples is required. Usually the excised tissue is fixed immediately after excision and 3D histology can be performed on the prefixed material. However, it has been shown to be advantageous to divide the tissue before as native, i.e., not-fixed material is smoother and therefore easier to flatten. The plane parts can then be fixed in formalin within the cassettes used for the routine paraffin embedding procedure. It is important to note that an orientation marker on the sample is absolutely vital (see Chap. 4 "Topographical Orientation") to aid in the later orientation of tumor outgrowths. It is advantageous to determine the top of the cassette as the position of 12 o'clock or of the earliest clock time.

Fresh Tissue Prepared for Formalin Fixation

The procedure starts with the placement of the now plane tumor margins (Fig. 3.2a) from the previously described

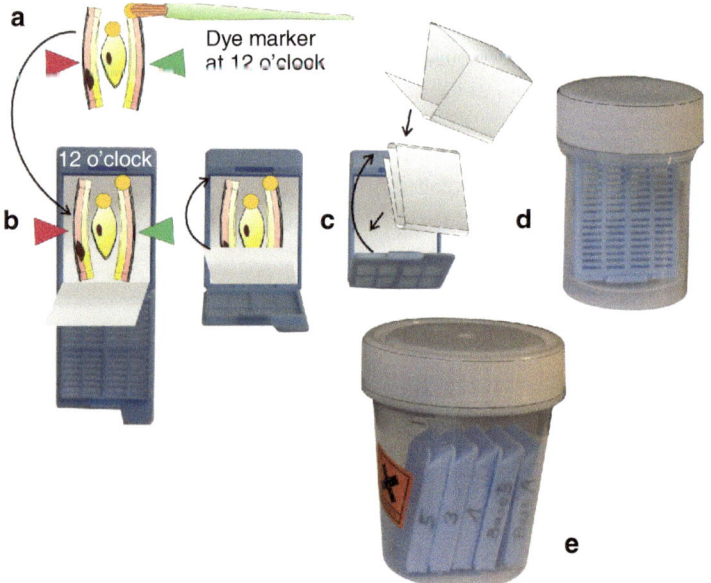

FIGURE 3.2 Fresh tissue prepared for formalin fixation in cassettes for paraffin embedding. Additional paper pillows to avoid torsion of tissue pieces

excisions (Chap. 2, Fig. 2.9) with their outside down into a standard cassette used for routine paraffin processing (Fig. 3.2b). The top of the cassette corresponds with the 12 o'clock position. If the specimen is very thin, pieces of embedding paper have to be added as a "cushion" to ensure tight closure of the cassette. This will flatten the underside of the tissue and avoid torsion of the tissue during the waxing process (Fig. 3.2c). The closed cassette is then placed into a small container with 4 % formalin fixation solution (Fig. 3.2d). If more tissue should be worked up, larger containers are available[1] (Fig. 3.2e). The tissue can be fixed either overnight at room temperature or for a fast fixation at 60 °C for 2 h. This short fixation time will be sufficient because the prepared tissue has a large surface and a small volume.

After fixation, the tissue will be dehydrated and paraffinized by a paraffinization robot in an overnight procedure and can be sectioned the next morning. After fast fixation, histopathological results are available after 20 h and after normal overnight fixation at room temperature after 32 h. Alternatively, tissue samples can also be shipped via courier services to the pathological laboratory for the diagnostic workup.

Embedding in a Mold with Paraffin

The embedding cassette with the now paraffinized tissue (Fig. 3.3a) is now opened while the lit has been removed (Fig. 3.3b). Then the tissue pieces are transferred into an embedding mold, pressing their outsides down (Fig. 3.3c, c'). It is crucial that the tissue is not flipped over, i.e., the orientation of the samples must stay the same. Now the embedding mold can be filled with liquid paraffin (Fig. 3.3d), and the bottom of the embedding cassette is pressed into the still hot paraffin as a lit (Fig. 3.3e).

---

[1]Langenbrinck Corp. www.langenbrinck.com;
e-mail info@langenbrinck.com

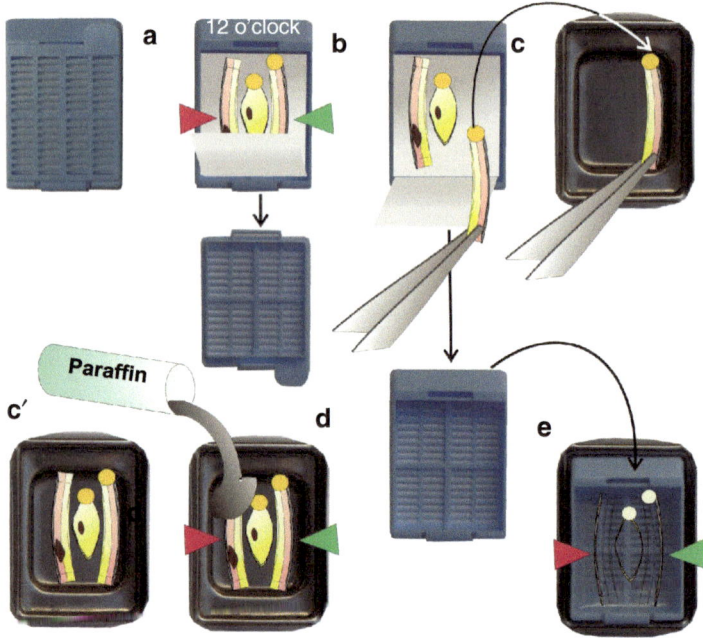

FIGURE 3.3 Embedding in a mold with paraffin to get a block for sectioning

Preparation of Paraffin Sectioning

The cooled and hardened paraffin block (Fig. 3.4a) has to be separated from the embedding mold by heating up shortly before the tissue can be sectioned in a microtome (Fig. 3.4b). The paraffin block with the embedded tissue will be strongly attached to the previously anchored embedding cassette and can therefore be used as a handle in the entire procedure. After removing the paraffin block from the embedding mold, the sample has to be flipped over and the plane outside of the specimens margins will point upwards (Fig. 3.4c, d) and clamped into the microtome (Fig. 3.4e). Please note the changing of the topographic orientation of the tissue margins

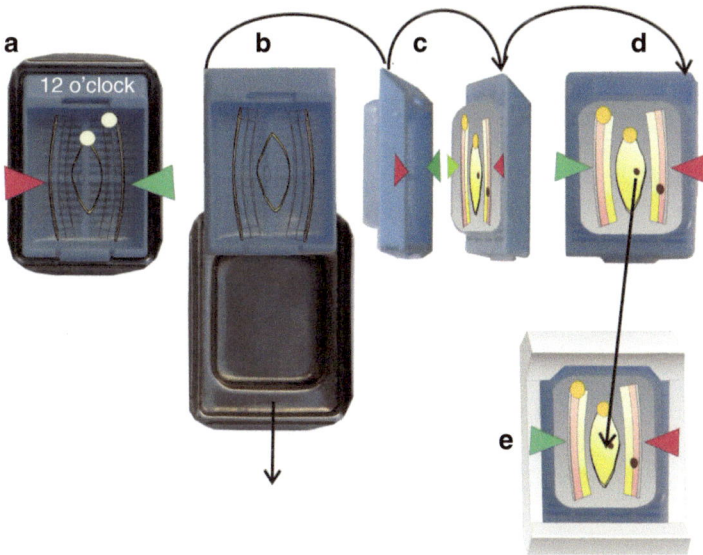

FIGURE 3.4 Preparation of paraffin sectioning flipping over the paraffin block, now showing the complete 3D outside of the specimen in a 2D plane

as a result of flipping over the block. The 3 o'clock position of the tissue margins will now be at the 9 o'clock position, and the outside of the margins will be on the surface of the paraffin block.

Paraffin Sectioning

After the paraffin block is clamped into the microtome, the sectioning of the tissue can begin (Fig. 3.5a). For best results, sections of 0.5 nm are recommended. Each section (Fig. 3.5b) is placed in a warm water bath (Fig. 3.5c). It is important not to change the orientation of the tissue during the transfer, i.e., the tissue should never be flipped over as this would change the orientation. The transferred paraffin section will float on

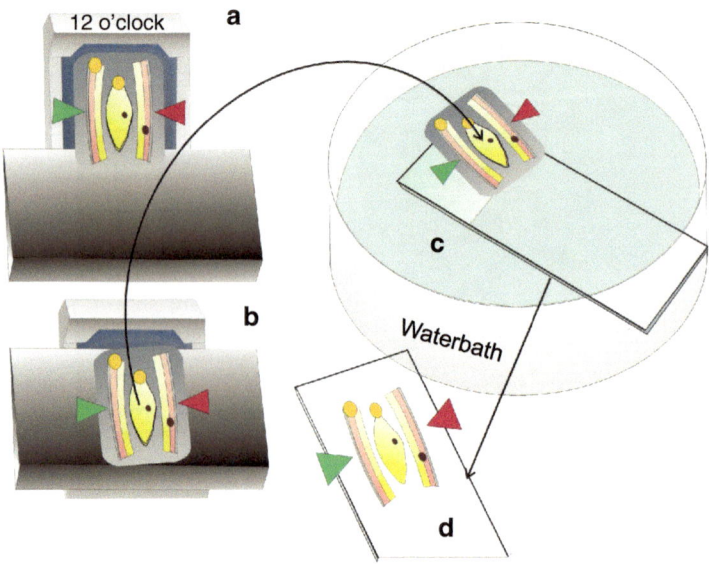

FIGURE 3.5 Paraffin sectioning. The paraffin sections are put carefully in a water bath and then from their backside on the slide

the water and can be moved onto a glass slide by moving the glass slide under the floating section in the water. The backside of the section will lie on the front side of the glass slide. Then the slide is moved out of the water with the paraffin section attached to it (Fig. 3.5c). To remove the wax of the slides, either Xylol or Histo-Clear® can be used. Then the slides are ready for H&E staining and the entire margins of the excised tumor can be evaluated in a full histological workup (Fig. 3.5d).

Division and Flattening of a Formalin-Fixed Tumor Specimen

As mentioned before, the margins and base of the excised tumor can also be prepared by a histopathological laboratory once the tissue has already been fixed in formalin [1].

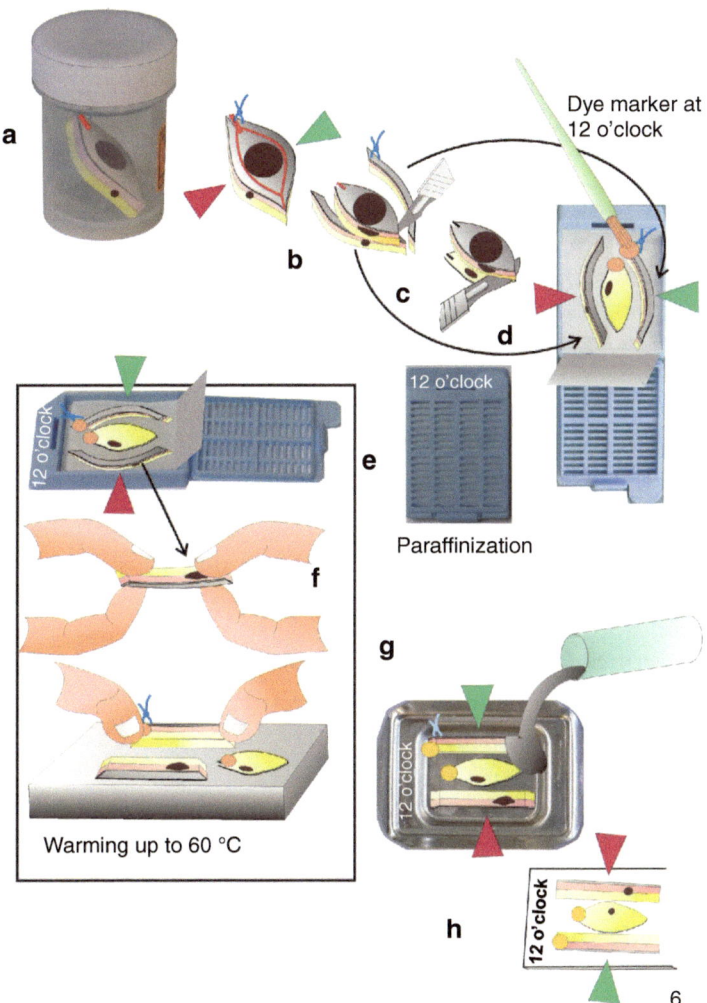

FIGURE 3.6 Preparation of a formalin-fixed tumor specimen. Flattening of the strips and base is possible if paraffinized tissue is warmed up

Much of the procedure follows the previously described preparation of native tissue (see figures in Chap. 2). However, as fixed material is less flexible than native tissue, some additional considerations in the process have to be taken into account.

The removal of the margin strips and bottom from prefixed tissue is done as previously described by cutting the margin and base of the excised tumor sample with a scalpel (Fig. 3.6a–c). This can be done easier with fixed tissue than with fresh tissue. But as prefixed tissue is more rigid than native tissue, the tissue cannot be properly flattened before it is embedded in the paraffin. However, this will not impair the embedding into paraffin. Therefore, prepared tissue margins and bottom of the sample are placed into an embedding cassette without fully flattening the samples (Fig. 3.6d) and embedded into paraffin using a paraffinization robot (Fig. 3.5e). Once the tissue is paraffinized, the waxy tissue is heated to 65 °C using an incubator. Then the tissue parts are removed from the embedding cassette and put on a heating plate. On the hot heating plate, the samples can be fully flattened with the outer side down almost as easy as native tissue (Fig. 3.6f). After flattening the tissue, the embedding and sectioning of the tissue can be done as previously described (Fig. 3.6g, h).

Cryo-sectioning

In a first and most critical step of cryo-sectioning, the 3D tumor sample has to be flattened to a plane with its outside down. As this is not easy, numerous methods have been developed in the past: Some of the methods use cooled metal cylinders; others use liquid nitrogen, freezing sprays, special clamps, or other devices. Here single-use commercially available standardized cryo-molds as shown in Fig. 3.1 will be used in the examples similar to the paraffin technique. These molds are easy to use and allow for standardized embedding procedure with clear rules that allow the separation of labor between different departments. As for the paraffin embedding procedure, the aim is to flatten the uneven excisional margins of the excised sample maximally to allow for a full histological workup.

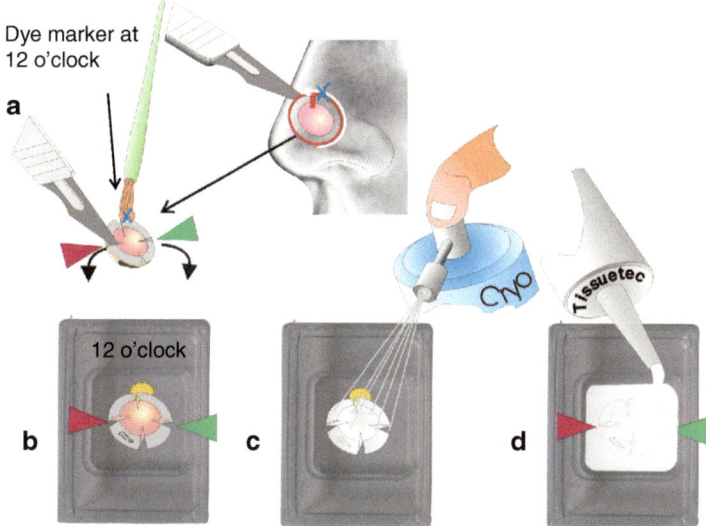

FIGURE 3.7 Embedding in a cassette for cryo-procedure using cryospray and Tissue-Tek

Embedding for Cryo-procedure

The excision of the tumor and its margins is most conveniently done with an oblique round excision resulting in the bowl-shaped tissue as described before (Fig. 3.7a or Fig. 2.1 for a detailed description). Then the flat tissue with the plane outside margins pressed down is frozen by a freezing spray or liquid nitrogen in a standard plastic mold (Fig. 3.7b, c). After freezing the tissue, the mold is filled up with cryogel which is frozen by liquid nitrogen or a freezing spray as described by the manufacturer (Fig. 3.7d).

Preparations for Cryo-sectioning

After embedding, the frozen block can easily be removed from the mold by heating up the outside shortly (Fig. 3.8a).

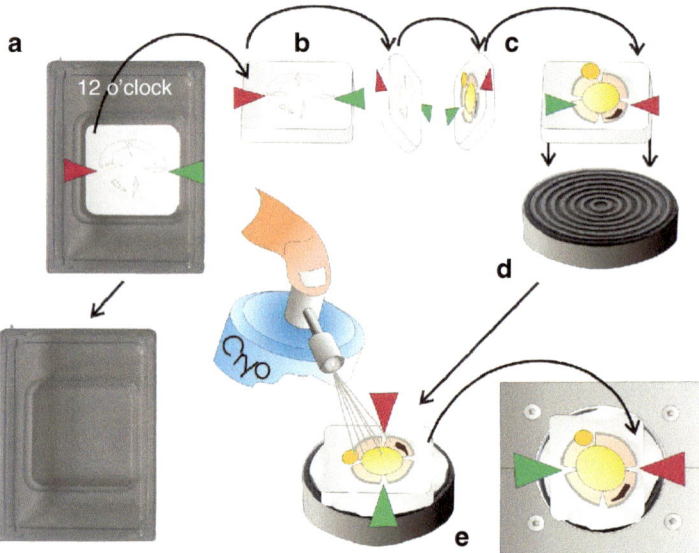

FIGURE 3.8 Preparations for cryo-sectioning flipping over the cryo block, showing the complete 3D margins of the specimen in a 2D plane

Then the block is flipped over, and the plane tumor margins will point upwards (Fig. 3.8b, c). The entire block can be attached to the tissue holder of a cryostat using cryogel and ice spray (Fig. 3.8d). This allows the plane margins to be sectioned (Fig. 3.8e). Please note the changing of the topographic orientation of the tissue margins as a result of flipping over the block.

Cryo-sectioning

The tissue that has been embedded in cryogel and attached to a tissue holder is now placed into a cryostat and sectioned (Fig. 3.9a, b). After each section of 0.5 nm, the tissue is taken up on a glass slide by pressing the front side of the slide onto the still frozen tissue (Fig. 3.9c). Each section

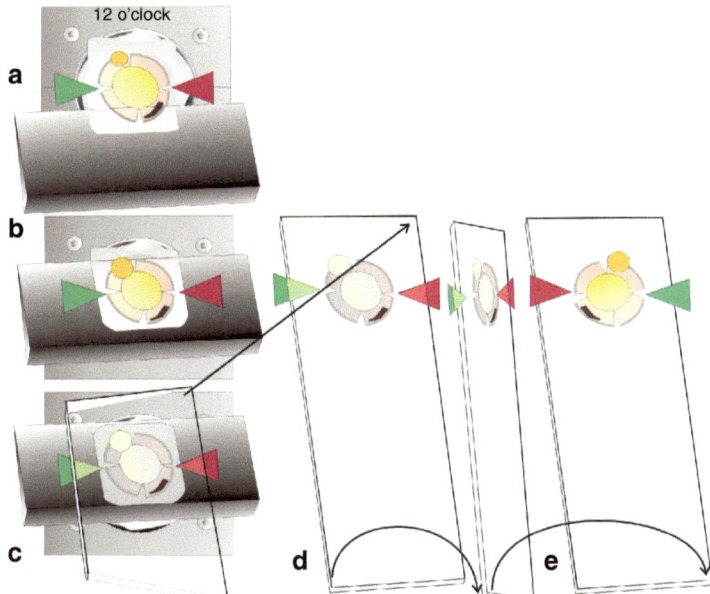

FIGURE 3.9 Cryo-sections are taken from their front side on the front side of the slide which will be then flipped over

should now represent the complete outside of the previously bowl-shaped specimen. The glass slide with the attached tissue is now flipped over to its front side (Fig. 3.9d, e) and can be stained with H&E (not shown). Note that after flipping the glass slide, the outside of the tumor specimen can now be seen in the original position relative to the patients defect.

Topographic Differences of Stained Histological Slides

After the margins of the tumor have been sectioned, a full histological workup has to follow. It is important to note that the topographic orientation of the slides differs between cryo- or paraffin sections due to technical differences in the

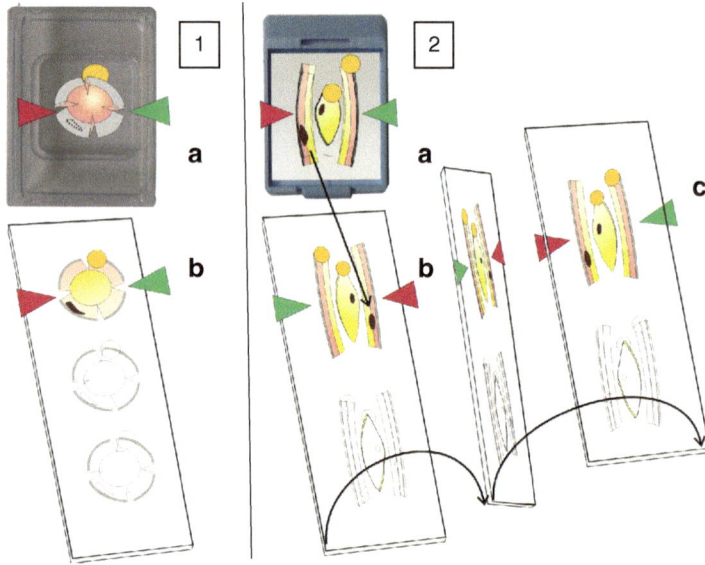

FIGURE 3.10 Topographic differences of stained histological slides: cryo-sections (*1*) show the view on the patient; paraffin sections (*2*) have to be flipped over to get the view on the patient. In the following figures, all paraffin slides are shown flipped over

procedure. Cryo-sections result in histological sections which can after the pathologist's investigation be directly projected onto the patients defect, i.e., these sections represent natural view to the patient's surface (Fig. 3.10, 1a, b). Three and 9 o'clock positions are identical. Paraffin sections on the other hand are always mirror-inverted images of the margins (Fig. 3.10, 2a, b), documented by the inverted 3 and 9 positions. Therefore, paraffin sections have to be turned over after the pathologist's investigation to allow a direct projection of tumor outgrows onto the patient (Fig. 3.10, 2c). This is because the top side of cryo-sections is taken directly from the knife of the microtome using the front side of the glass slide (Fig. 3.9c), whereas paraffin sections are first moved to a water bath and then taken from below up to the front side of the slide (Fig. 3.5d).

Due to the technique of sectioning, the first few sections of either cryo- or paraffin sections in most cases do not represent the whole plane of the excised tumor. Therefore, multiple, deeper sections into the tumor are necessary until the whole plane of the embedded specimen is encompassed. Usually 3–6 sections are necessary, in some cases even more. Depending on the size of the sections, two or three of them are put on one slide. The deeper the sections, the better tumor outgrowths can be seen. Even if not the entire plane of the tumor is represented in a section, it is recommended that all sections are preserved on slides to allow for a full histological analysis of the tumor excision. In our experience, it has been proven useful to place the first section on the top of the glass slide. Consecutive sections will follow until the first full section which will usually be localized at the bottom of the slide. To investigate the sections, the pathologist first analyses the last and deepest (nearest to the tumor) section. This section normally covers the entire outside of the incision and should be representative and of best quality. Therefore, tumor outgrowths are seen here at best and easiest. If tumor outgrowths are found in this section, three interpretation possibilities have to be distinguished.

Possibilities for Evaluation of Complete or Incomplete Excision

In the first example (Fig. 3.11, 1) shown here, a tumor outgrowth is found between 6 and 9 o'clock in the last and deepest section (nearest to the tumor) (Fig. 3.11, 1a) and in the first, very superficial section as well (Fig. 3.11, 1b). In this case, a re-excision at the position between 6 and 9 o'clock has to be done.

In the second example (Fig. 3.11, 2), tumor parts which are found between 7 and 8 o'clock in the last and deepest section (Fig. 3.11, 2a) are found in the consecutive section but not in the first and most superficial section in which this part the margin is fully represented (Fig. 3.11, 2b). In this case, the full

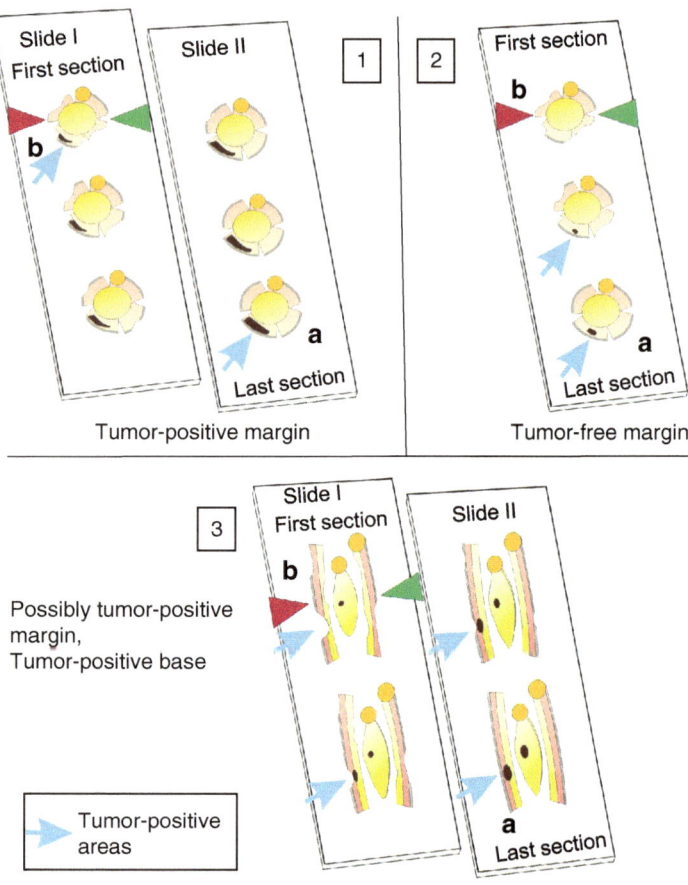

FIGURE 3.11 Possibilities for evaluation of complete or incomplete excision with the first and the last section towards the tissue center, rsp. tumor

tumor outgrowth was contained within the margins of the excised sample, and no re-excision would be necessary. For this diagnosis, it is absolutely pivotal that a full consistent stretch of healthy tissue is represented at the position of the tumor outgrowth in the first section.

In the third example (Fig. 3.11, 3) in the deepest section, tumor outgrowths are detected at 8 o'clock within the lateral margin and central towards 9 o'clock in the base (Fig. 3.11, 3a), but the first section shows a lack of tissue at the position at 8 o'clock of the margin (Fig. 3.11, 3b). Here the containment of the tumor outgrowth cannot be verified, and re-excision has to be done for the safety of the patient. Artifacts like this can happen quite frequently as the first sections often do not encompass the full margin of the tumor.

Reference

1. Breuninger H, Schaumburg-Lever G. Control of excisional margins by conventional histopathological techniques in the treatment of skin tumours. An alternative to Mohs' technique. J Pathol. 1988;154: 167–71.

Chapter 4
Dividing Tumors and Topographical Orientation

So far only on examples of small tumors in which the excised tumor specimen fitted completely in the device for histological sectioning were discussed. If tumors are larger due to their advanced growth or larger safety margins, the resulting specimen may not fit completely onto the devices used for histological sectioning. In these cases, the excised specimens have to be divided in parts small enough to be sectioned by either cryo-sectioning or paraffin sectioning raising new complex issues of topographical orientation which will be discussed in the following.

Guideline for Dividing Tumors

The principal technique of 3D histology can be used for all sizes of tumors. However, in larger-sized tumors the topography of the 3D histology becomes more complex. The division of the excised tumor can be done in several ways, much to the liking of the surgeon and/or the pathologist. Important and common for all divisions, however, is that the 3D margin of the tumor is divided in a way allowing for a full 2D representation. Thickness and size should be suitable for processing. The diameter of the tissue is usually limited by the embedding procedure, i.e., cryo-sections have to be smaller than paraffin-embedded sections (Table 3.1). The thickness of the tissue which has to be embedded should be 2–4 mm. Also, in

H. Breuninger, P. Adam, *3D Histology Evaluation of Dermatologic Surgery*, DOI 10.1007/978-1-4471-4438-0_4, © Springer-Verlag London 2013

all instances the divisions have to allow for a full reconstruction of the 3D margin. Otherwise, a precise localization of the tumor outgrowth on the patient will be impossible to achieve. Therefore, it is vital to mark division planes not to lose orientation for required re-excisions.

As mentioned before, also the choice of oblique or vertical excision technique influences the way how the tumor is divided. The separation of the tumor margins and dividing in parts fitting for further processing has to be done by the surgeon or pathologist as shown in Chap. 2. In the following these different methods, including important methods for topographic orientation, will be illustrated and discussed with examples for mid-sized and large tumor excisions.

A common feature for all large tumors is that topographic matching of the borders will be proportionally more difficult the larger the tumors are grown. Or in other words, the larger the tumor, the higher is the need of an exact topographic orientation of the tissue. The results can be illustrated also by schematic of drawings or in terms of clock times (i.e., with a marker at 12 o'clock in relation to the axis of the body), thus making topographic orientation easier. Digital photographs may be helpful.

Topographical Orientation

A combination of fixed rules and dye dot markers can greatly facilitate the orientation. The best experiences were made with simple embedding rules using the aid of a clock division for orientation (Table 4.1). Here each piece is assigned to a certain time relative to its position, i.e., 3 o'clock marking the farthest right and 9 o'clock the farthest left position of the tumor excision and 12 and 6 o'clock the top and bottom, respectively. If the 12 o'clock marker (suture or incision) is placed relative to the top of the patient's head, a very good orientation of diagnosed tumor outgrowths on the patient can be maintained. However, depending on the localization and kind of excision, e.g., spindle-shaped excision, it might be useful to slightly deviate from these rules by placing the 12

TABLE 4.1 Rules for topographic orientation

1. 12 respectively 0 o'clock suture marker or deep incision in direction to the patient's top of the head.

   In case of re-excision always planning one clock time more than the tumor positive extension at the margins is described. The marker always is set at the earliest clock time. If the re-excised margin begins, e.g., at 9 o'clock until 4 o'clock, this means 9 over 12–16 o'clock. The marker is set at 9 o'clock.

2. Division of the margin in pieces and the base in a clockwise order in equal sizes from right to left like the hand, fitting in the cassettes for histopathological procedures.

3. In case of first excision, the suture marker remains at the right side of 12 o'clock in direction to 1 o'clock.

4. Embedding of the first margin strip in a cassette at the right side, epidermis to the right. The earliest clock time of the strips lies always at the top of the cassette beginning with 12/0 o'clock.

5. The next strip at the left side, epidermis to the right, earliest clock time to the top.

6. In case of two strips within the cassette, only the strip on the right side gets a marker at its earliest clock time to avoid exchange errors.

   In case of re-excision the second strip on the left gets two markers, one at the earliest clock time and a second in the middle.

7. Pieces of the base get a marker at the earliest clock time of the circumference as well (usually only one piece in a cassette).

8. In case of small tumors only two strips can be put in the natural view into one cassette, first strip right side, epidermis to the right and second strip on the left side, epidermis to the left, of both 12 o'clock position at the top.

9. In complex locations and large tumors, additional suture markers at the defect margin, drawings, or photographs of the site are necessary.

o'clock positions relative to the top of the spindle, for example. In these cases it is very important to thoroughly document these deviations from the rule in the patient's chart.

Sutures have to be removed before sectioning. Therefore, it will be necessary to maintain the orientation by other means. As the standard paraffin embedding cassettes have a defined top and bottom side, the orientation of the cassette can be used to maintain the orientation of the tissue. If the top of the cassette is defined as 12 o'clock, the risk of misunderstandings can be avoided. Furthermore, it is recommendable to standardize the loading of the cassettes. The margin strips should always be put from right to left in the clockwise order beginning with the right side of the cassette and epidermis always the right. If these rules are strictly followed, mixups can be excluded.

Some might find the usage of dot markers to be of help in keeping track of the topographic orientation within the 3D margins. Even though such markers might not be necessary if the tissue loading is highly standardized, they are recommendable and do help to avoid exchange errors. Easy-to-handle markers are correction fluids such as "Tipp-ex®" (Table 4.2).

Besides strict embedding and division rules, there are also a number of histological dye markers available which can be used for topographic orientation of tissue samples. Choosing a color for each side of a division can be helpful for orientation after sectioning. Most dye markers commonly used will be visible after tissue processing and staining for histological

TABLE 4.2 Dye markers

Dye marker for drawing excision lines on the skin:

Eosin solution in 98 % isopropyl alcohol which is used for skin disinfection

A fine clamp can be used as a pen

Histological marking colors:

Green, blue, orange, black

WAK – Chemie Medical GmbH Steinbach Germany www.wackchem.com

A good and simple alternative for black:

TIPP-EX (R) fluid

Société BIC F- 92611 Clichy Cedex, France www.bicworld.com

diagnostics. Therefore, these markers have one additional advantage: Sometimes the entire specimen is not represented in one section (see Fig. 3.11). If color markers are used, it is less likely that these instances are missed, as the full section will always be colored at its entire margin. This additional safeguard may also improve diagnostics. However, strict embedding rules, routine, and experience of the pathologist will lead to the same result, and the processing time will decrease significantly.

In conclusion, the complexity of topographic orientation always requires special protocols and clear rules. Setting markers by incisions or sutures, the embedding routine, drawings, and dye markings are all important aids for orientation and can be used either individually or in combination depending on the preference, experience, and expertise of the involved parties. As a rule of thumb, it should be remembered that the larger the tumor, the more effort is needed for marking and dividing whichever method is used.

In the following sections the handling of different-sized tumors will be discussed in detail. For each tumor size several excision, division, tissue processing, and topographic marking rules are illustrated. The combinations are not mutually exclusive and are solely chosen to simplify the description of the entire variability of available methods. It should be emphasized that a full 3D histological workup of the tumor margins can be achieved in several ways.

Handling of Tumor Specimens of ca. 2 cm Diameter

In the previous chapter, different kinds of excision and methods of flattening the borders of the margin were discussed independently. In the following examples of the procedure from excision, dividing the tissue and the conversion from 3D margins to a 2D plane for histology is shown. As discussed before the tumor can either be removed together with the safety margins in one step and divided later or the clinical visible tumor and the margins are removed in consecutive excisions. However, it is advantageous to cut out the tumor by a knife and not by curettage to make the histological investigation easier.

Dividing an Excised Specimen into Two Parts (Oblique Excision, Cryo-sectioning)

Similar to the excision of smaller tumors, the first step here is the removal of the tumor proper for diagnosis using curettage (Fig. 4.1a). Now the marker at the 12 o'clock position is set. In this example an additional suture (violet) is set at the patient's site to facilitate later orientation. Then the tumor "shell," i.e., the margin is removed in a 360° oblique excision resulting in a bowl-shaped defect (Fig. 4.1b) and specimen (Fig. 4.1c). Larger tumors of ca. 2 cm diameter usually have to be divided in two parts to fit for cryo-sectioning, and a dye

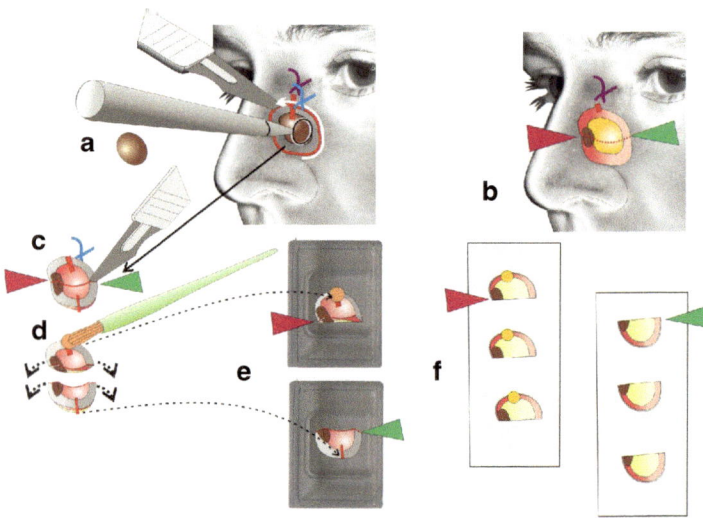

FIGURE 4.1 Dividing an excised specimen, too large for one cassette into two parts. Embedding in cryo-cassettes and resulting histological slides

marker is set at 12 o'clock (Fig. 4.1d). The divided parts can be flattened in one plane with some further cuttings and placed into the cryo-embedding mold with their outside down (Fig. 4.1e). Now both parts are processed as described before and the final H&E-stained histological slides will represent the entire 3D exterior of the tumor which can be examined for tumor outgrowths (Fig. 4.1f). As the example shown here uses cryo-sectioning, the orientation of the sample is the same as on the patient seen in comparison to the defect (see Fig. 3.10, 1). A simple dot marker at a defined position, here at 12 o'clock, is absolutely sufficient to avoid orientation errors. As mentioned before, more dye markers might help later in the orientation of the divided tumor margins.

Dye Marking of All Margins to Ensure Correct Orientation (Oblique Excision with Cryo-sectioning)

Rather than excising the tumor margins in one 360° incision, the parts of the margins can also be excised in independent excisions. Some might find it helpful for later orientation to mark the division plane on the patient prior to the excision of the two parts, e.g., at 3 and 9 o'clock with two stitches as shown (Fig. 4.2a). The two turned pieces can now be marked using

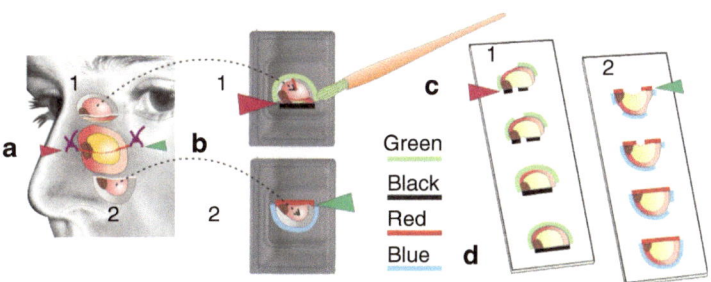

FIGURE 4.2 Dye marking of all margins to ensure correct orientation and complete margins

different colors before cryo-sectioning. While the outer circumference of the upper part is marked in green, the lower part is marked with blue. For the easiest reconstruction of the tumor, it might be useful to also mark the division line in other colors, e.g., black and red (Fig. 4.2b). Now the fully marked specimens are sectioned and after H&E staining inspected for tumor outgrows. As the colors will be visible in the sections, they can be used to help orientation (Fig. 4.2b, c) and representation of the specimen on the slide. As the first sections, neither in cryo-sections nor in paraffin embedded tissue, represent the whole plane of the tissue, the margins will not be fully colored (Fig. 4.2c). Deeper sections are necessary until the margin color is present in the whole plane of the embedded specimen (Fig. 4.2d, see also Fig. 3.11). Therefore, the staining helps to determine the depth of the sections until the entire margin is covered.

Dividing an Excised Specimen into Two Margin Strips and Base (Vertical Excision, Paraffin Embedding)

The differences between oblique and vertical excision have been discussed previously and it remains to the individual surgeon which excision technique is preferred (see Chap. 2 for details). If a vertical excision is preferred, it is usually better to remove the tumor with the safety margin before dividing it up (Fig. 4.3a). However, the clinical tumor can be excised in a first step as shown in Figs. 2.3 and 2.5. The 12 o'clock marker is placed in the beginning. After the excision the margin strip of 2–3 mm is cut from the specimen in one consecutive strip using the 12 o'clock mark as starting point (Fig. 4.3b). The cut strip (12–12 o'clock) can be flattened with its outside down. To fit the entire outside margin in embedding cassettes, it has to be divided in two smaller fitting parts (12–6 and 6–12 o'clock). A 12 o'clock suture marker at the beginning of the strip is replaced by a dye dot (Fig. 4.3c).

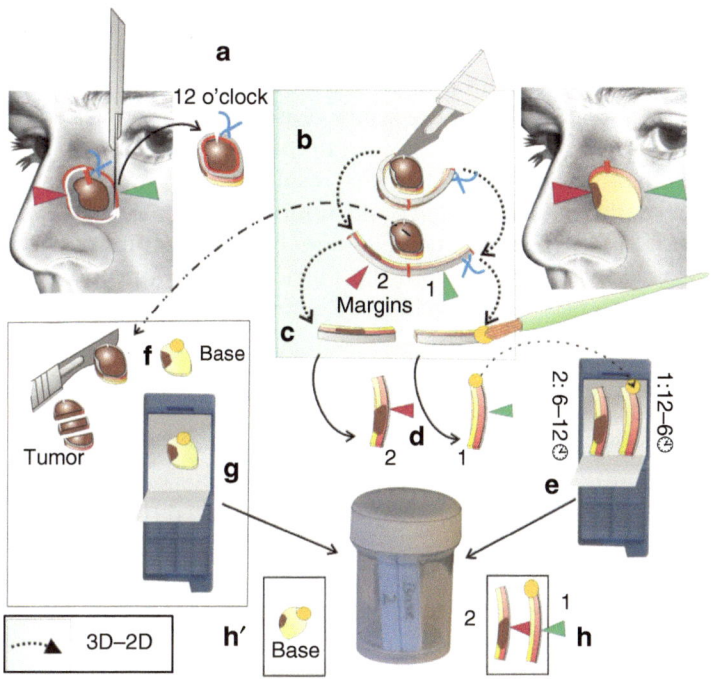

FIGURE 4.3 Dividing a tumor in two margin strips and base, embedding in paraffin cassettes following a rule and resulting flipped over histological slides

To place the pieces into the embedding cassettes, some rules should be followed to facilitate topographic orientation. First the pieces of the margin are turned 90° (Fig. 4.3d) and placed into the cassette with the outside of margin facing down. It is important to fill the cassette always in the same order and orientation, e.g., clockwise from the right to the left with the epidermis facing to the right. Following this rule, the first strip (12–6 o'clock) would be placed at the right side, epidermis to the right, and the 12 respectively. 0 o'clock position, i.e., earliest, at the top of the cassette. The following strip (6–12 o'clock) would be placed to the left of the previous again with the earliest clock time (here 6 o'clock) at the top of the cassette (Fig. 4.3e). If this rule is always followed, mix-ups and confusion can be fully avoided.

Now the bottom (base) of the remaining tumor specimen is removed and also marked at its 12 o'clock position (Fig. 4.3f). The remaining central tissue is used for tumor diagnostic. The base and also parts of the tumor center can now be placed in a second cassette (Fig. 4.3g, cassette on the left). After fixation, embedding and sectioning the resulting slides will represent the entire outside margin of the tumor, and after H&E staining they can be investigated (Fig. 4.3h, h'). As paraffin sectioning was used in this example, the outside is now flipped over to image the view to the patient (explanation see Fig. 3.10, 2).

Handling of Tumor Specimens of ca. 3 cm Diameter

The larger the tumor, the more differentiated the dividing of the tissue will be. The next examples explain the procedure step by step in case of a middle-sized tumor for oblique and vertical cutting. Despite the large size, even bigger tumors can be removed in one piece and divided later. It is also possible to remove the margins consecutively in several excisions as it was shown before. However, as the complexity of the divisions is now increasing, special handling rules and additional dye markers are necessary for the orientation after processing. In the following several scenarios of handling mid-sized tumors are described in detail.

Dividing a Tumor into Four Parts on the Patient (Oblique Excision, Cryo-sectioning)

If the margins are excised step by step on the patient, the tumor should be removed first by curettage or excision (Fig. 4.4a). Beginning at 12 o'clock, the margins are then excised in parts fitting for cryo-sectioning indicated here as red lines (Fig. 4.4b, 1, 2). Following a clockwise order, the next parts are excised (Fig. 4.4c). For topographic orientation, each tissue part should be marked with a different dye at each side or alternatively by a dye dot marker only at the side

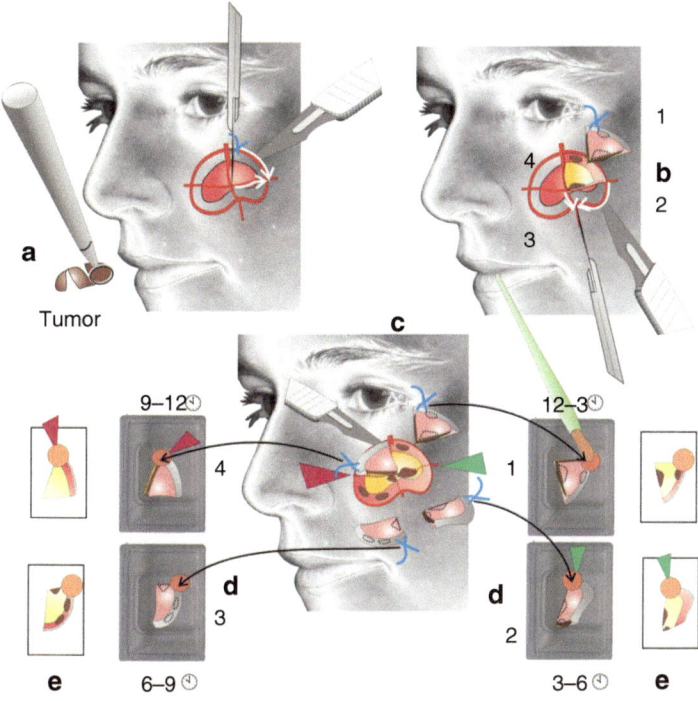

Tumor

FIGURE 4.4 Dividing a tumor in four parts. Embedding in cryo-cassettes with a rule and resulting histological slides

facing the previous excision, i.e., at its "earliest" position at the outer border following the clock (Fig. 4.4c). Now the divided pieces can be put in the embedding mold following the clockwise order (1 = 12–3/2 = 3–6/3 = 6–9/4 = 9–12 o'clock, Fig. 4.4d). The marker and epidermis define the orientation for each piece in the histology (Fig. 4.4e).

Dividing a Tumor in Three Margin Strips and Base (Vertical Cutting, Paraffin Embedding)

After placing a marker at the 12 o'clock position (optional at the patients site), the tumor is removed with the subcutaneous tissue and a safety margin by a vertical cut (Fig. 4.5a).

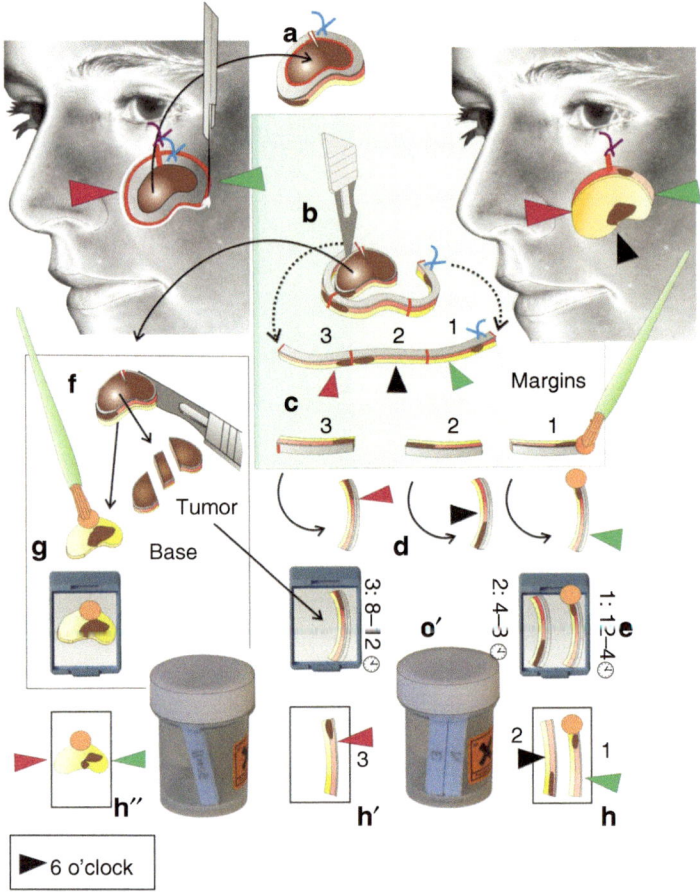

FIGURE 4.5 Dividing a tumor in three margin strips and base, embedding in paraffin cassettes with a rule and flipped over histological slides

Then the margin is separated from the tumor in a strip of 2–3 mm as described before (Fig. 4.5b). The strip is pressed flat with its outside down and for later topographic orientation a dye dot marker is set left at 12 o'clock on the margin (Fig. 4.5c). The strip is divided into equal pieces fitting in the standard embedding cassettes and turned 90° (Fig. 4.5d). The flat three margin parts (1 = 12–4 o'clock, 2 = 4–8 o'clock, 3 = 8–12 o'clock) are put into the cassettes (Fig. 4.5e, e′) following the previously mentioned rules, i.e., in clockwise order from right to left with the "early" time point towards the top and the epidermis to the right. In this way the outside of the margin will be facing down as it is required for sectioning, and the margin with the 12 o'clock marking will be the farthest right part with the marker at the top (Fig. 4.5e). Now also the left and right strips cannot be mixed up in the cassette containing only two margin parts. The third strip is placed in another cassette again in clockwise order (Fig. 4.5e′).

Then the bottom of the specimen is cut away (Fig. 4.5f) and the remaining tissue is used for tumor diagnostic. If it is useful the tissue of the tumor could be placed within the same cassette of the third margin strip. Due to the different nature of the parts, these parts cannot be confused and therefore no further dye markings are required. For later topographic orientation, a dye dot marker has to be set at 12 o'clock on the base (Fig. 4.5g). The base is taken in the last cassette; here the previously placed 12 o'clock marker will be sufficient for orientation (Fig. 4.5h). After fixation, embedding and sectioning the resulting slides are seen in mirror-inverted orientation if paraffin embedding was used, to show the tumor outgrowths in the view on the patient (Fig. 4.5h, h′, h″).

Handling of Very Large Tumors of ca. 4 cm and More Diameter

In large tumors the investigation of the complete tumor boarders is very important as the number of outgrowths statistically increase with the size of the tumor. Normal histopathological methods with vertical serial sections (See Chap. 9) have larger gaps in larger tumors, nevertheless needing a high effort. These gaps will lead to a higher rate of recurrences as the results are often false negative. Using 3D histology also on very large tumors will allow for a full investigation without gaps and can secure a complete tumor excision. Here first an oblique excision followed by cryo-sectioning is illustrated. This is followed by a demonstration of a vertical excision using paraffin embedding. While in smaller tumors the differences between these two alternatives have not been apparent, in tumors of very large size, the effort will be notably reduced. As before, the combinations oblique excision with cryo-section and vertical excision with paraffin embedding are freely interchangeable and are only chosen to simplify the demonstration. The principal handling of very large tumors for 3D histology is not much different compared to mid-sized or small tumors. Only the fact that the margins of larger tumors are also larger adds complexity to the excision of this size of tumors.

Dividing a Large Tumor into 11 Parts (Oblique Excision, Divided on the Patient, Cryo-sectioning)

As before, the tumor is excised first with oblique cut (Fig. 4.6a). After the removal of the tumor, the margins have to be isolated in a second oblique excision. However, due to the size of the tumor, the margin has to be divided to fit for further processing. In the example shown here, the margin is divided as described by the red lines (Fig. 4.6b). This division can be done on the patient by several independent excisions. Markers are set using clock times as dividers for a circle, always the earliest time of each tissue and at 12 o'clock at the base. Some might find it also helpful to set markers on the patient as well before dividing the tumor (the different colors of the markers are not necessary in reality). In this case a suture would be placed at each red line in Fig. 4.6b. Alternatively the division of the specimen can be done after the removal of the entire margin. Depending on the size of the tumor, quickly a large number of margin parts have to be handled, here eight margin parts (Fig. 4.6c) and three parts of the base (Fig. 4.6d). In Fig. 4.6c the suture markers will be replaced by dye dots to allow sectioning. Similarly the three base parts of the tumor can be marked each with only one dye (Fig. 4.6d). After the careful marking of the excisions, the tissue is now processed and sectioned using cryo-sectioning (Fig. 4.6e, e') and can then be examined histologically (Fig. 4.6f, f').

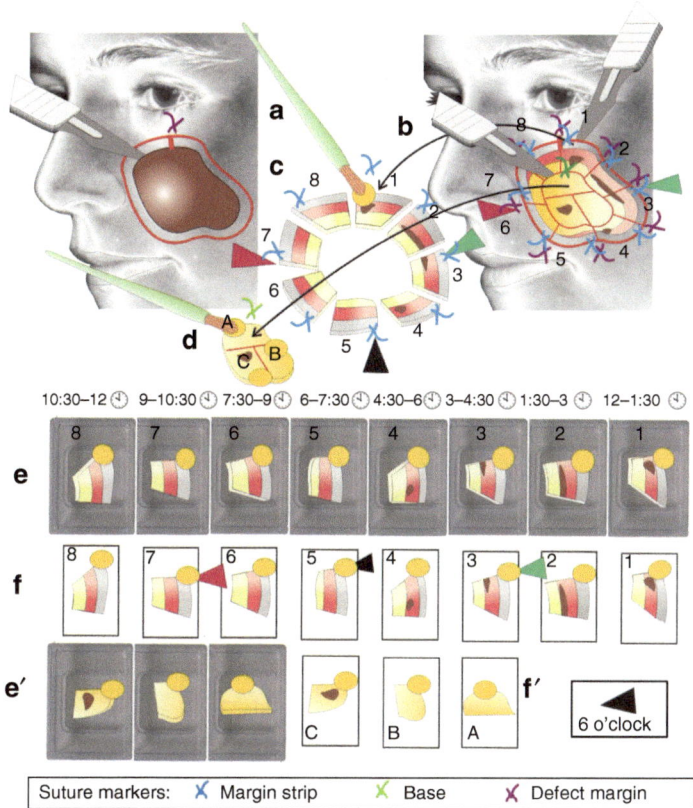

10:30–12 🕐 9–10:30 🕐 7:30–9 🕐 6–7:30 🕐 4:30–6 🕐 3–4:30 🕐 1:30–3 🕐 12–1:30 🕐

| Suture markers: | ✗ Margin strip | ✗ Base | ✗ Defect margin |

FIGURE 4.6 Dividing a tumor into 11 parts of the margin and of the base, embedding in cryo-cassettes with a rule and histological slides

Dividing a Large Tumor into Eight Parts of Strips and Base (Vertical Excision, Paraffin Embedding)

Larger tumors excised by a vertical incision follow the same basic procedures. As always, the procedure should start by placing a 12 o'clock marker. Then the tumor including the safety margin is excised as previously described. After the excision the lateral margin strip of the specimen of 3–4 mm

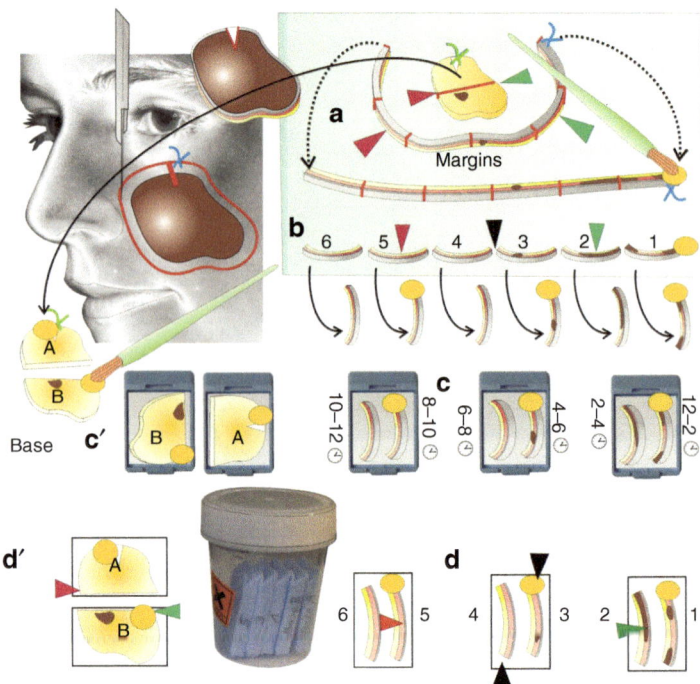

FIGURE 4.7 Dividing a tumor into eight parts of margin strips and base, embedding in paraffin cassettes with a rule and flipped over histological slides

in width is separated from the excised specimen starting at the 12 o'clock position in one continuous cut. The suture marker at the beginning point at 12 o'clock is replaced by a dye marker (Fig. 4.7a). In order to isolate the full margin, the basal tissue of the tumor has to be isolated separately.

For large tumors the margin strip will be relatively long and has to be divided for further processing. Instead of using several dyes for orientation, a time-logic can be applied to keep track of the relative position of tumor outgrowths found later. Time-logic, tissue structure, and strict embedding rules within the cassettes allow a full reconstitution of the 3D tumor margins. In this method the tumor strip is divided in parts representing several sections of a clock. Depending on the size of the tumor, the number of pieces can differ considerably up to one for each hour or more if necessary. In the example shown here, the tumor is divided in six pieces each representing a 2-h section of a circle (Fig. 4.7b). Then all pieces are turned 90°, pressed flat with the outside of the tumor margin facing down and the epidermis facing to the right. Now all sections are placed in embedding cassettes by loading the samples clockwise from *right to left* like the hand. Three cassettes are needed. To avoid confusion about the orientation of similar looking tissue samples, each right most strip can be marked using a dye at its top or "earliest" clock position (Fig. 4.7c). The base is divided in two parts with dye markers and embedded as well (Fig. 4.7c′). After sectioning the resulting H&E-stained slides will be in a mirror-inverted orientation to show the natural view on the patient (Fig. 4.7d).

Similarly to the margin usually the base of the tumor has to be divided like in the example shown here in two parts or more depending on the size of the tumor. However, in order to use the limited space of the embedding cassettes most efficiently, the rule of placing the 12 o'clock position of the tissue towards the top of the cassette should be broken here. For the tumor base it is recommendable to turn the samples and place those longitudinally into the cassette (Fig. 4.7c′). Here the previously placed 12 o'clock marker and other markers at the "early" time points, i.e., 3 o'clock as shown in the example here, will allow for sufficient orientation in the histological sections even if the rule was changed. If this procedure is followed, it is sufficient to simply turn the histological slides to return to the original orientation on the patient after possible tumor outgrowths have been diagnosed (Fig. 4.7d′).

Using time-logic rather than dyes might need some time to get used to. However, if strictly applied this method usually will be quicker, reliable, and equally thorough compared to methods using dyes. Furthermore, the time-logic has the advantage that each piece automatically will get coordinates relative to the head of the patient. Therefore, localization of the outgrowth for required re-excisions will be easy.

In conclusion, the number of variations to divide tumors is staggering and here only some examples were introduced. The basic principle in all surgical procedures is the same and exchangeable. As long as the entire tumor margin is isolated and analyzed, there are no clinical differences. However, healing rates and complications can be very different depending on the method used. Therefore, it is up to the personal preference of the surgeon which technique or which combination of methods is used. Equally important for all methods is the introduction of topographic mapping rules and their strict compliance by all persons involved.

Mapping Surgeries in Case of Unclear Margins

There can be cases where the border of the tumor is not clearly defined or where the tumor has infiltrated sensitive areas in the face like nose, eyelids, or ears. In these cases a full excision of the tumor might not be recommendable in the first instance as too much tissue would have to be removed leaving difficulties in closing the defects with minimal scaring. Therefore, it might be advisable to do an exploratory surgery first to determine the full margins of the tumor. In this way a more targeted and therefore minimal invasive excision can be done. After this initial exploratory surgery, a more targeted surgical procedure can be planned in order to remove all tumor parts.

There are essentially two ways to map the boundaries of a tumor. One method is to take multiple punch biopsies of the surrounding area (Fig. 4.8a). To be able to map the biopsies back to the patient, they should be taken according to a previously drawn map or in a clockwise order around the tumor (Fig. 4.8b). The disadvantage of this method is that tumor infiltrations might be missed as relatively large gaps are introduced. To avoid this issue and if it is planned to remove the tumor anyway, the entire tumor margins also can be isolated before the final excision in a minimal invasive procedure.

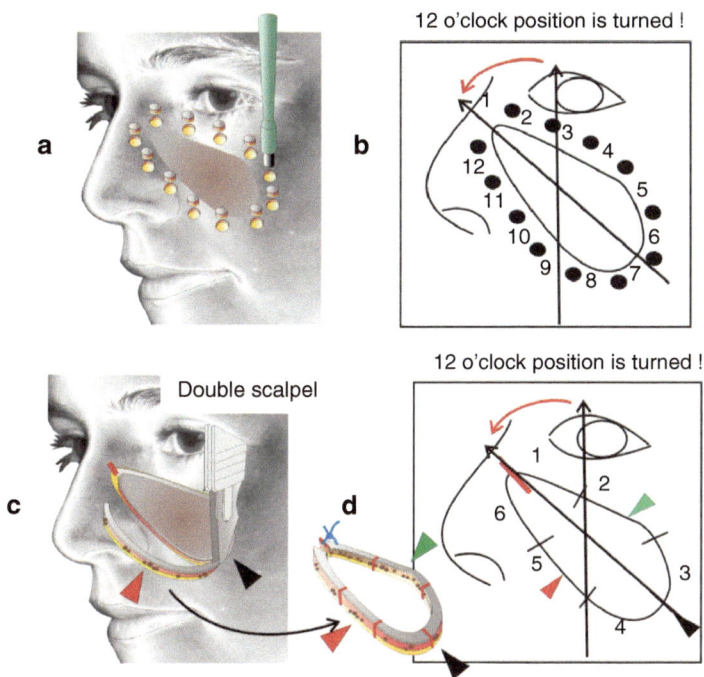

FIGURE 4.8 Mapping operations in case of unclear margins with punch biopsies or a margin rim only. Twelve o'clock position is changed due to anatomical practical considerations

Using a double scalpel (putting two scalpels with a bandage together), the margin sometimes can be isolated more easily by a cut along the assumed margins of the tumor (Fig. 4.8c). The tumor and its base are then removed in independent procedures either together or after each other. The excised margin can be evaluated as previously described using 3D histology. In this way a complete map of the tumor can be drawn without the risk of introducing gaps. As always in this kind of surgeries, it is absolutely vital to maintain a topographical map.

These maps can be adjusted in special tumor configurations or localizations so that the smallest amount of healthy tissue has to be removed. As shown in the two examples, it might be helpful to turn the 12 o'clock position according to the longitudinal axis of the specimen (Fig. 4.8b, d). However, it is important to clearly document such changes sufficiently in the patient's chart like in the shown example where 12 o'clock responds to the back of the nose.

Chapter 5
Communication with the Lab

The General Procedure (Workflow)

The management of a full 3D histology needs a tight communication between the surgeon and the pathologist. Clear and safe rules are necessary to enable both the surgeon and the pathologist to point out areas of incomplete tumor excisions very precisely. In Mohs' micrographic surgery, the surgeon and pathologist is the same person. This has advantages because a communication with other institutions is not necessary.

However, it is difficult to have a high level of surgical and pathological skills in one person despite some training courses. On the other hand, a good communication with strict rules allows the cooperation between two specialized institutions. In the beginning, these specialists should come to an agreement which dedicates parts of the procedure to each person or department. Considering the complexity of the procedure, a number of different workflows are imaginable. In general there are following steps to consider (see Fig. 5.1):

Workflow Between the Surgeon and the Histopathological Lab

Some of these steps will be allocated to one department by their nature. Of course, the excision and re-excisions of the tumor will always be done by the surgeon. It is also sensible

H. Breuninger, P. Adam, *3D Histology Evaluation of Dermatologic Surgery*, DOI 10.1007/978-1-4471-4438-0_5, © Springer-Verlag London 2013

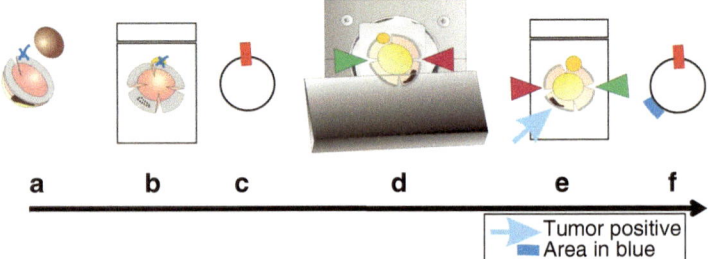

Tumor positive
Area in blue

FIGURE 5.1 Workflow between the surgeon and the histopathological lab. (**a**) Excision and re-excision of the tumor and margins. (**b**) Conversion of the 3D margins into a 2D specimen ready for sectioning and documentation. (**c**) If useful, a map of the topographic situation. (**d**) Tissue embedding and sectioning. (**e**) Preparation of histological slides and diagnostics. (**f**) If useful, a map of tumor-positive areas

to assume that the pathologist will be responsible for producing the cryo-sections or paraffin sections and the diagnostics. After that, however, it is possible that the pathologist or the surgeon divide the fresh tissue and prepare the conversion of the 3D margin into a 2D slide. For orientation an incision is sufficient if the surgeon performs the division, flattening, and embedding of the tissue; a suture is necessary if the pathologist does this.

It is also possible that the tissue is always fixed and the pathologist will work with prefixed material only (Table 5.1). What way of collaboration is chosen depends on the local conditions. In any case, the communication and documentation between the different institutions involved have to include data of the patient, diagnosis or assumed diagnosis, localization, the size of the visible tumor, and the taken safety margin.

Communication with a Form

The most important tools for communication between different departments are strict rules and communication regulations (Table 4.1), with the help of a form and, if useful, maps,

TABLE 5.1 Workflow between surgeon and pathologist. Five possibilities

	Surgeon or assistance	Pathologist or assistance
1.	Surgery and histopathology one person	
2.	Surgery and division of the fresh tissue, embedding in cassettes for histopathological processing. Examination of the slides as well for topographic information	Sectioning, staining, and examination of the slides
3.	Surgery and division of the fresh tissue, embedding in cassettes for histopathological processing	Sectioning, staining, and examination of the slides. Topographic information
4.	Surgery and marking fresh tissue pieces, each in a wet compresse and written on for the lab	Division of the fresh tissue for histopathological processing. Sectioning, staining, and examination. Topographic information
5.	Surgery and marked fixed tissue to the lab	Division of the fixed tissue for histopathological processing. Sectioning, staining, and examination. Topographic information

drawings, or photographs. Here the most important regulation is the communication of topographic orientation marks using clock times as a grid. This will make the reconstruction and communication of tumor-positive findings in most cases relatively easy as shown in an example form in Fig. 5.2.

With this system a picture or drawing will not be necessary in cases of straightforward, smaller tumors. It is sufficient to communicate solely by using clock times for orientation purposes. In principle the same communication can be also used in cases of larger tumors. If the surgeon prepared the samples for histology, all relevant topographic information should be transferred to the pathologist (Fig. 5.2a). Using a circle as representation of the separation between tumor base and margin (Fig. 5.2b), the pathologist can point out the exact position of an outgrowth by referring to different positions on the circle in clock times, here between 7 and 8 o'clock (Fig. 5.2c). This system will be sufficient to point out tumor outgrowths.

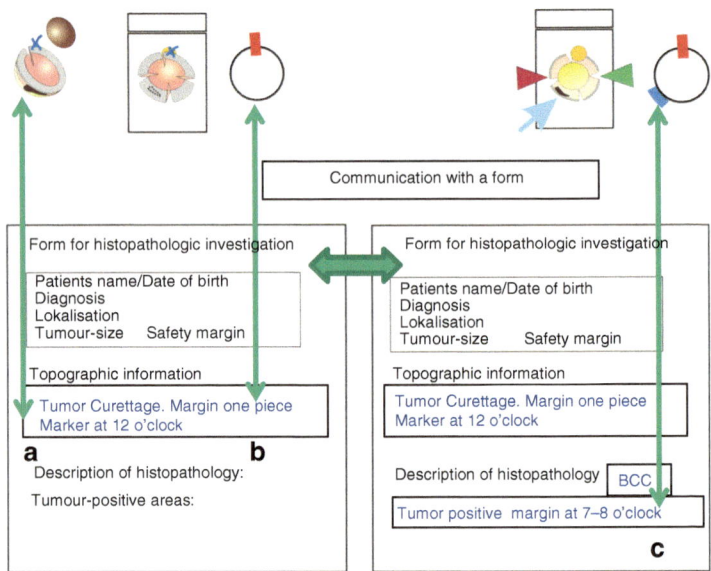

FIGURE 5.2 Communication between the surgeon and the lab with a form

The advantage is that it is very simple to communicate and easy to implement in any electronic communication.

Documentation and Information Exchange Within the Workflow of 3D Histology

This section discusses the information exchange within the previously described workflow in respect to the conversion of the 3D tumor margins into 2D histological sections and back to the 3D defect. By using the clock-based documentation of tumor outgrowths, it is possible to convert pathological findings on the 2D slide to the respective 3D margin on the patient. In the following the basic principles of good practice documentation will be introduced using first examples of small tumors prepared by either oblique or vertical excisions.

These basic principles are then used in examples of larger tumor excisions where the documentation is slightly more complex due to the increased number of specimens which have to be analyzed. The examples here always use drawn maps for a better understanding. However, it should be noted that due to the simplicity of the clock-based orientation system, these maps are only necessary in larger and complex tumor specimens.

As previously described the standard workflow in the 3D histology can be divided into several subsections. It is important that each step is well documented and easy to understand to avoid confusion. To simplify the steps in the following five examples, the workflow is reduced to four steps:

(a) Division of the tumor margins.
(b) Topographical situation (description with clock times or/ and with a map).
(c) Embedded parts of the margins and the resulting histological slides with detected tumor-positive areas. The view on both is similar with one difference only: The embedded tissue is seen from above within the cassette, while the slide shows the plane underside representing the outer margins (see Chaps. 3 and 4). *Up to now one schematic figure shows both views together.*
(d) Communication of the tumor-positive areas topographically (description with clock times or/and with a map).

Mapping of Tumor-Positive Areas and Re-excision, Two Cassettes (Tumors of Figs. 4.1 and 4.3 Cut for 3D Histology in Different Ways)

In the examples shown here, the basic principles for good practice documentation are illustrated using an oblique (Fig. 5.3 row 1) or vertical (Fig. 5.3 row 2) excised tumor specimen. When the tumor is excised, it is recommendable to give exact data of clock times or to draw a map of the excised tumor indicating the most important hallmarks of the tumor such as the 12 o'clock position and the division

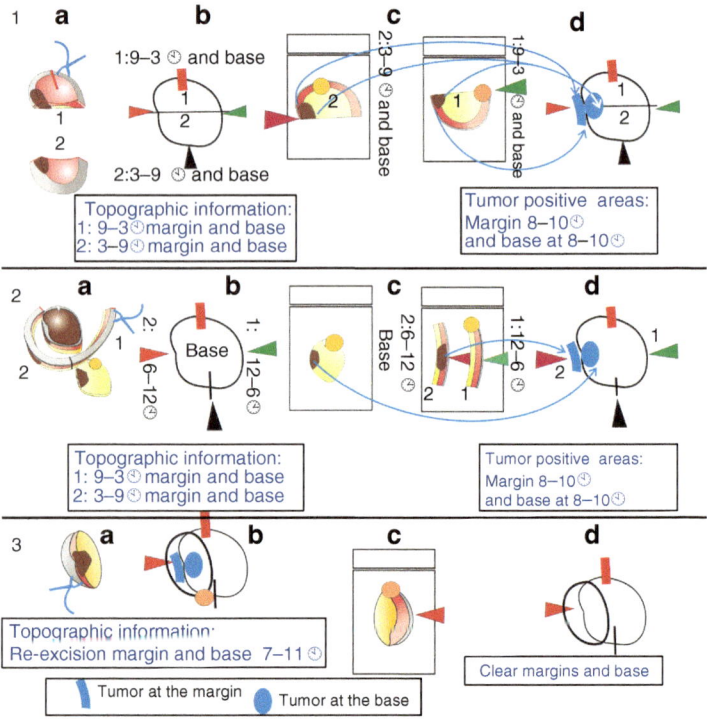

FIGURE 5.3 Mapping of tumor-positive areas at a tumor, cut for 3D histology in different ways (*1* and *2*). Re-excision at tumor-positive areas (*3*)

plane (Fig. 5.3 column a). In the case of the oblique excised tumor, a division plane at the smaller diameter in the middle (3–9 o'clock) would be sufficient to get pieces for embedding (Fig. 5.3 column a row 1). Topographic information is given by clock times (piece one 9–3 and piece two 3–9 o'clock) or with the aid of a map. In the case of a vertical excision, the tumor will most likely be divided by separating the margin in the described clockwise manner and the base in independent samples. The topographic information is given in clock times as well (12–6, 6–12 o'clock and base) (Fig. 5.3 column b row 2).

The now divided tumor samples will be embedded (Fig. 5.3 column c) and sectioned both seen in the above described view together in one. Tumor outgrowths, visible after H&E staining, are shown in blue (Fig. 5.3 column c). Depending on the division or excision method, histological slides will look differently. In the oblique excision tumor margin and base are in one piece on two slides (Fig. 5.3 column c row 1), and in the vertical excision tumor base and margin will be on independent slides (Fig. 5.3 column c row 2). Using the previously produced maps, these findings can easily be marked in the respective areas (Fig. 5.3 column d) or/and have to be written down using the clock scheme. In the example here this would be tumor positive at the margin 8–10 o'clock and base 8–10 o'clock. As oblique and vertical excisions produce the same results, there are no differences in the diagnostics (Fig. 5.3, column d, row 1 and 2).

In this way it will be easy for the pathologist to refer the findings onto the documentation with the correct topographic orientation of the tumor outgrowths. In the same time it will also be easy for the surgical team to locate these findings on the patient in the next re-excision. The surgeon gives the information to the pathologist: Re-excision from 7 to 11 o'clock together with the base (Fig. 5.3 row 3a, topographic information row 3b). The tissue is embedded with the described rules (epidermis to the right and the earliest clock time above, Fig. 5.3 row3c) and sectioned. The histological findings are clear margins (Fig. 5.3 row 3d). For more details see Chap. 6.

The system of marking tumor outgrowths by clock times and maps might seem a little complicated especially in larger tumors. However, once it is fully understood, it is very intuitive and easy to follow and allows for a straightforward conversion of the 2D results of the pathologist into the 3D margin of the defect. If all involved people are used to this system of rules for topographic orientation (Table 4.1), the workflow between surgeon and pathologist (Table 5.1) will be facilitated. To illustrate the full potential of this system, more variations with larger tumors will now be illustrated.

Mapping of Tumor-Positive Areas of a Larger Tumor, Four Cassettes (Tumor of Fig. 4.4, Oblique Excision)

Also for larger tumors the communication with clock times or/and a map will facilitate the communication between all people and departments involved in the procedure. Here the tumor is divided in four specimens (Fig. 5.4a), which are shown together with clock times and on a map but indicated by the division lines (Fig. 5.4b). After embedding and sectioning and staining, the pathologist can now bring the individual pieces back into their original order and mark the detected tumor outgrowths on the map. The tumor-positive areas are transferred onto the map as indicated by the blue arrows, i.e., tumor outgrowths in the center should be indicated in the respective position within the circle and outgrowths found in the margin on or outside of the circle (Fig. 5.4c). This map can then easily be communicated to the surgeon using the clock time scheme. Here this would be

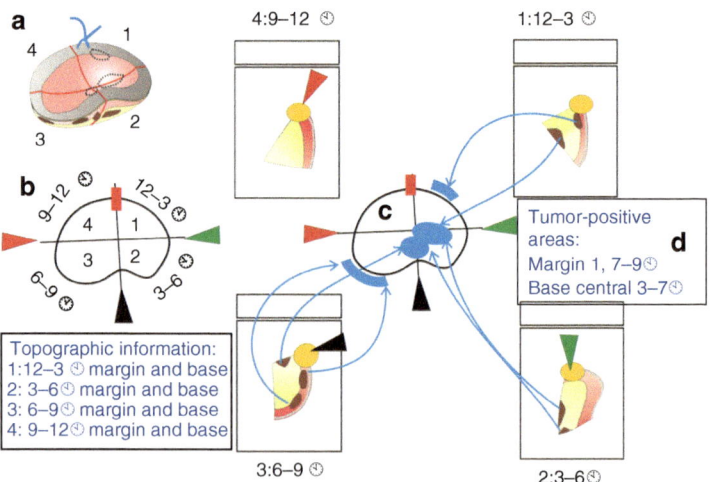

FIGURE 5.4 Mapping of tumor-positive areas at a larger tumor, oblique cut using four cassettes (tumor see Fig. 4.4)

margin positive at 1 and 7–9 o'clock, base positive central, and towards 3–6 o'clock (Fig. 5.4d).

Mapping of Tumor-Positive Areas at a Larger Tumor, Three Cassettes (Tumor of Fig. 4.5, Vertical Excision)

In this example the tumor specimen has been divided in four parts as well but in another shape: three margin strips from 12 to 4 o'clock, 4–8 o'clock, and 8–12 o'clock and one base (Fig. 5.5a). As before, clock times or/and a map indicating all divisions can be given to facilitate the communication (Fig. 5.5b). After sectioning the pathologist can now easily transfer the findings onto the map. For better understanding of this step, the tumor margins of the slides are shown here also in topographical orientation. Using this mental reorientation, the tumor outgrowths can now be easily drawn onto the map (Fig. 5.5c). Also in here the information for the surgeon can be communicated using the clock scheme; here this

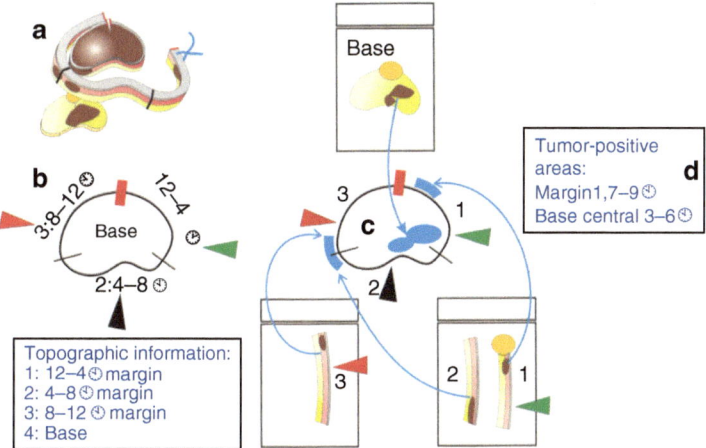

FIGURE 5.5 Mapping of tumor-positive areas at a larger tumor, vertical cut using three cassettes (tumor see Fig. 4.5)

would be margin positive at 1 and 7–9 o'clock, base positive central, and towards 3–6 o'clock (Fig. 5.5d).

Mapping of Tumor-Positive Areas at a Very Large Tumor, 11 Cassettes (Tumor Fig. 4.6, Oblique Excision)

Very large tumors have to be divided several times, which makes orientation slightly more complicated. Here the tumor has been divided in 11 parts: 8 margin strips and 3 parts of the base (Fig. 5.6a). To allow the pathologist orientation of the tumor pieces, all divisions should also be shown on the map (Fig. 5.6b). Using this map the pathologist will be able to bring

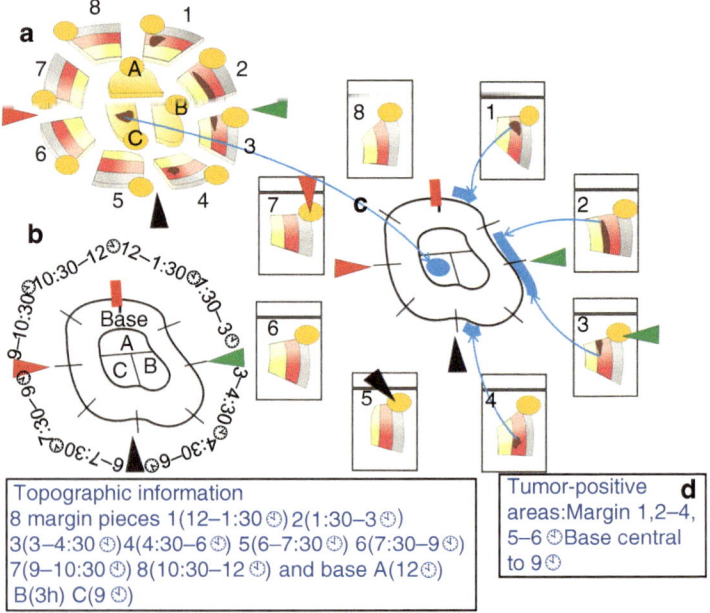

FIGURE 5.6 Mapping of tumor-positive areas at a very large tumor, oblique cut using 11 cassettes (tumor see Fig. 4.6)

the individual sections into the correct order and transfer the findings onto the map (Fig. 5.6c). Also in this case the information for the surgeon can be easily communicated using the clock scheme, which makes the map almost obsolete. Compared to a relative complex drawing, the same information can be communicated by margin positive 1, 2–4, and 5–6 o'clock, base positive central, and towards 6–9 o'clock (Fig. 5.6d).

Mapping of Tumor-Positive Areas at a Very Large Tumor, Five Cassettes (Tumor Fig. 4.6, Vertical Excision)

If the sample is excised vertically and paraffin procedure is used, usually less divisions of the tumor will be required. Here the tumor has been divided in 8 parts: 6 margin strips and 2 parts of the base (Fig. 5.7a). Nevertheless, it is highly

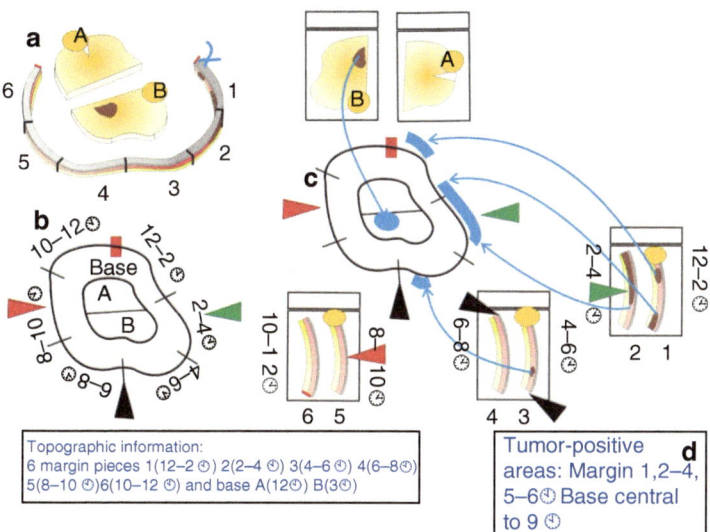

Figure 5.7 Mapping of tumor-positive areas at a very large tumor, vertical cut using five cassettes (tumor see Fig. 4.6)

recommendable to document all division planes thoroughly as clock times or/and onto a map to allow the pathologist to orientate all specimens correctly (Fig. 5.7b). After sectioning the pathologist will have to reorientate all margin parts according to their original position in his/her mind. After this mental transition of the margin parts, the findings can now easily be transferred onto the drawn map (Fig. 5.7c). Using the clock orientation scheme, the finding could also be translated to margin positive at 1, 2–4, and 5–6 o'clock, base central, and towards 6–9 o'clock (Fig. 5.7d).

Taken together, this chapter shows that the communication between pathologist and surgeon can be relatively easy and clear if simple rules are followed. The workflow can be organized and with comprehensive documentation misunderstandings can be avoided. If there are uncertainties or if the localization of the tumor does not allow a straightforward simple excision, additional documentation such as maps and/ or photographs are highly recommendable (see Chap. 6). After the diagnosis of the pathologist, the surgeon now has to transfer the findings onto the patient, which will be discussed in the next chapter.

Chapter 6
The Aftermath or How to Excise Until Clear Margins

As we have seen in the previous chapter, topographic landmarks facilitate the precise localization of tumor-positive outgrowths in the entire 3D margins. With the help of this information, the surgeon can then carry out accurate topographic resection of these areas to completely remove the tumor. In these resections it is again important to topographically mark the tissue so that any further tumor-positive areas at the incision margins can be detected. Due to the potential complexity of this procedure, tumors might have more than one outgrowth so multiple samples will be taken; it is again imperative to set up some rules for marking the individual resections (Table 4.1). First for safety reasons for these re-excisions, it is recommendable to start the incisions always at the position corresponding to 1 h earlier as the diagnosed positive outgrowth and to end 1 h later. The safety margin depends on a lot of factors which are discussed for the first excision in Chap. 8 (see Table 8.3). Most important; small margins in sensible locations and if single clock times are positive; larger, if a lot of clock times are positive and if too much re-operations should be avoided. In the face normally the margin width will be between 2 and 8 mm. In the depth usually one layer deeper is taken. Second it is recommendable to set the markers in a clockwise order, starting always at the position of the earliest time of the clock of the first/previous excision. If tumor outgrowths reach, e.g., in one area

H. Breuninger, P. Adam, *3D Histology Evaluation of Dermatologic Surgery*, DOI 10.1007/978-1-4471-4438-0_6,
© Springer-Verlag London 2013

from 9 to 4 o'clock passing 12 o'clock (that means 9–16 o'clock), the 9 o'clock position will be the earliest. The resection starts at 8 o'clock (here the marker is set) and ends at 17 o'clock. Every independent re-excision gets an extra marker at the earliest clock time. It may be useful to set suture markers at the patient to mark the re-excision area or to allow later correct orientation.

Embedding the tissue pieces into the cassette, it may be advantageous to place two independent re-excisions into one embedding cassette. Since all isolated strips of the re-excision get a marker at the earliest clock time, the second one (left side of the cassette) should be marked twice to avoid confusion. The tumor base sample should always be marked at the relative 12 o'clock position of the primary excision. This process is repeated until complete removal of the tumor is ensured. In the following the full excision of tumors will be discussed in several examples of re-excisions using various surgical methods. As before, it is important to note that the choice of method is freely exchangeable to the liking of the executing surgeon.

Re-excision Using 1. Oblique Excision (Tumor Examples of Figs. 4.4 and 5.4) and 2. Vertical Excision (Tumor Examples of Figs 4.5 and 5.5)

Here the required re-excisions of the previously excised tumor examples shown in Figs. 4.4, 4.5, 5.4, and 5.5 will be discussed. The shown tumors were excised using either an oblique or a vertical incision technique. As shown in Chap. 5, both of these tumors show tumor outgrowths at various positions making a re-excision of these areas necessary.

Using the documented positions for orientation, the tumor-positive areas are now removed using either an oblique (Fig. 6.1, 1) or a vertical (Fig. 6.1, 2) incision. In the examples shown here, the tumor outgrowths were diagnosed at 1 o'clock and 7–9 o'clock at the margin (Fig. 6.1, 1b, 2b). Therefore, the

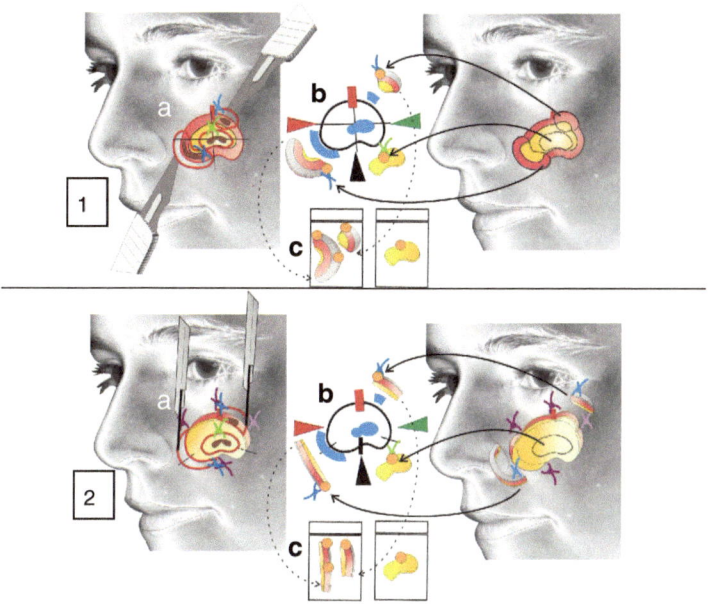

FIGURE 6.1 Re-excision (1): Oblique excision (See Figs. 4.4 and 5.4) (2): Vertical excision (See Figs. 4.5 and 5.5)

re-excisions should be placed from 12 to 2 o'clock and 6–10 o'clock, respectively. Suture makers are placed at the earliest clock times of the removed margin strips. Similarly the positive outgrowths at the tumor base should be excised with the next deeper layer and a generous margin of usually 3–6 mm lateral and a suture marker at 12 o'clock (Fig. 6.1, 1a, 2a). In example (Fig. 6.1, 2) optional suture markers are set at the patient to allow further orientation. For better visualization the re-excised tissue parts are shown here at their relative topographic orientation (Fig. 6.1, 1b, 2b, note the larger sample compared to the diagnosed outgrowth). For embedding and sectioning, the epidermis should always be placed to the right and the outer margin down, bringing the early position for both samples to the top of the cassette (Fig. 6.1, 1c, 2c). Also, the re-excised specimens should be marked at their earlier position relative to the clock division of the primary excision, i.e., at 12 or 6 o'clock (Fig. 6.1, 1c, 2c). In case two independent re-excisions are placed into one embedding cassette, the second strip is marked twice to avoid confusion. The tumor base sample should always be marked at the relative 12 o'clock position of the primary excision (Fig. 6.1, 1c, 2c). In the case shown here, the histological workup is negative and no further re-excisions are required. However, sometimes multiple re-excisions are required. One example of such a tumor will be discussed in the next figure.

First and Second Re-excision of a Large Tumor (Vertical Excision, Tumor of Figs. 4.7 and 5.7)

In this example tumor-positive outgrowths were found at position 1, 2–4, and 5–6 o'clock and at the central area of the base as discussed in Fig. 4.6 and shown in the map of Fig. 6.2a. Following these findings the affected areas have to be removed using again a vertical incision. For safety reasons it is again important to include larger sections of the margin by placing the incision at the position corresponding to 1 h earlier and 1 h later of the finding, which in the example shown here leads to one large re-excision from 12 to 7 o'clock of the lateral margin (Fig. 6.2b, shown here in its original topographic orientation for better understanding). The suture marker is inserted at the earliest clock time at 12/0 o'clock. In the re-excision of the base marked at 12 o'clock, already muscular tissue can be reached as indicated by the purple color. After re-excision the samples are divided and placed from right to left with the epidermis to the right and the outside down into the embedding cassette (Fig. 6.2c). For topographic orientation of these connected margin strips, the first tissue strip should be marked at its earliest time point relative to the original first excision or, in the case of the tumor base, at 12 o'clock (Fig. 6.2c). It is helpful to turn the 12 o'clock position of the base fitting better in the cassette according to the longitudinal axis of the specimen.

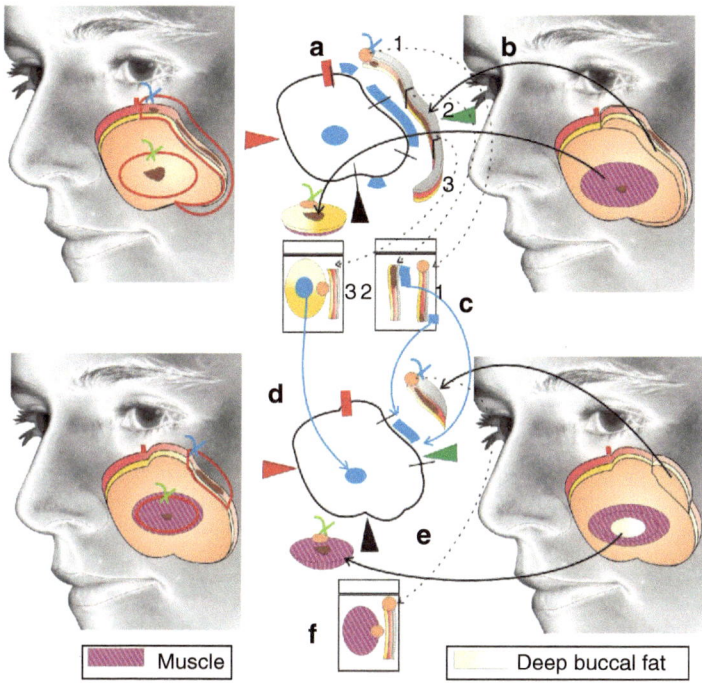

FIGURE 6.2 First and second re-excision of a very large tumor vertical excision (See Figs. 4.7 and 5.7)

As in the example shown here in Fig. 6.2c, further tumor outgrowths were found in the margin at 2 o'clock and the central base (Fig. 6.2c, d). Therefore, a second re-excision has to be made at the respective areas again with a safety margin of one clock time in either direction, i.e., from 1 to 4 o'clock with its marker (Fig. 6.2d, e). Due to the deep outgrowth at the central base position, even tissue underlying muscular tissue can be reached, as shown in this example by reaching the buccal fat (Fig. 6.2e). As the size of the re-excisions is decreasing with repetition, now both re-excised specimens will fit in one embedding cassette (Fig. 6.2f). This process should be repeated until no tumor-positive areas can be found, as shown here in Fig. 6.2f.

As a general rule, it should be noted that for safety reasons re-excisions at the margins and the base have to be done always generously. If this procedure is followed until no tumor-positive tissue is found in the histological sections, the rate of local recurrences will be very low.

In many cases of smaller-sized tumors, the defect of the first excision was closed immediately after the excision by primary suturing, as the probability of tumor outgrowths in these cases is below 50 %. However, if after the 3D histology workup of these excised smaller-sized tumors shows outgrowths, re-excisions will be required even if scars have formed already. Under consideration of the closing method, tumor-positive sides can be mapped and re-excised to the respective position relative to the scar, perhaps again with an immediate reclosure after the re-excision. Also in cases where the primary defect was closed using skin flaps or skin transplantations, a targeted re-excision will be possible as long as all margins have been analyzed using 3D histology. But this needs special experience.

Scar Re-excision After 3D Histology and Primary Wound Closure (Positions of Outgrowths Are Known)

In the previously described example of a spindle-shaped tumor excision (Fig. 2.10), the 3D histology revealed positive outgrowths at the lateral margin between the positions 7 and 8 o'clock and at the base at 9 o'clock (Fig. 6.3a). However, the defect was closed immediately. The orientation of the scar can be used for orientation in order to position the re-excision correctly. Depending on how the defect was closed, the scar will mark the 12–6 o'clock axis and it will be therefore easy to remove tissue from the scar from the margin at 6–9 o'clock including corium and subcutaneous tissue. Due to the diagnosed outgrowths at the base, the 9–10 o'clock excision cut should include also deeper muscular tissue (Fig. 6.3b). This rather small excision can be closed again immediately. The outside of the tumor outgrowth containing tissue has to be brought into one plane by placing several length- and crosswise cuts and marked at its earliest time point for orientation (Fig. 6.3c). It can be embedded and analyzed further (Fig. 6.3d).

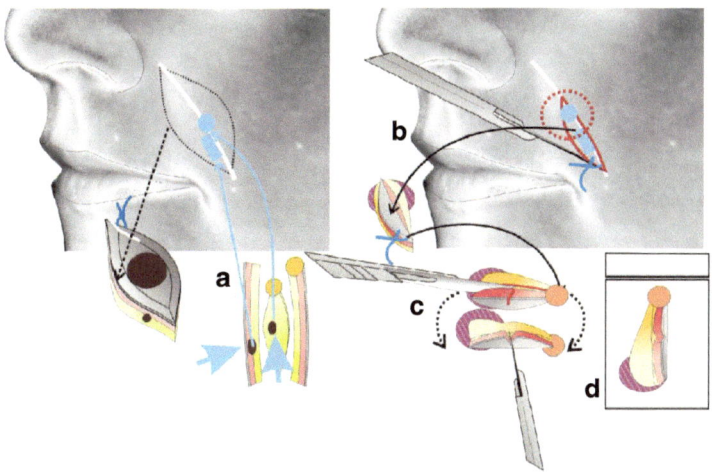

Figure 6.3 Scar re-excision of tumor-positive margin and base together after 3D histology and primary wound closure (See Fig. 2.10, spindle-shaped excision)

If the primary excision was done without the use of topographic markers or if after scar formation due to other circumstances, no precise localization of identified outgrowths is possible, the positions of outgrowths has to be determined by the removal of the entire scar. Here it is important to remove all scar tissue including a lateral safety margin and a layer of deeper tissue beneath the scar formation. The removed scar can then be analyzed using 3D histology to determine the outgrowths secondarily.

Scar Re-excision After Primary Wound Closure (Position of the Remaining Tumor Is Not Known)

If scar tissue has formed already after the primary excision of the tumor and tumor-positive areas were found, the entire scar including a safety margin and deeper laying tissue beneath the scar has to be removed. In cases of smaller scars, the excised tissue can then be separated along the scar and flattened with

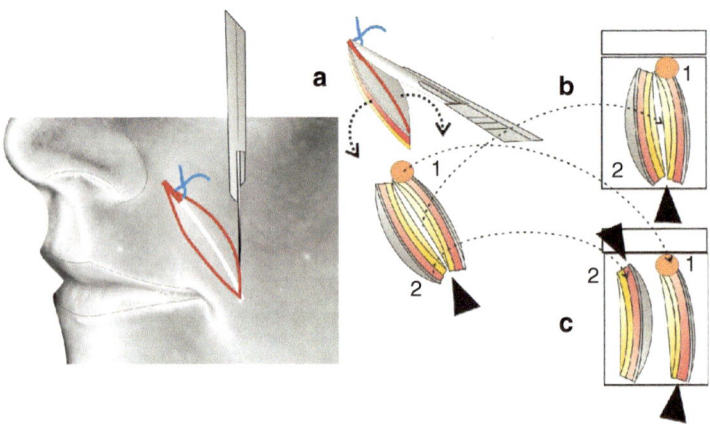

FIGURE 6.4 Scar re-excision after primary wound closure. Position of the remaining tumor is not known

the outside facing down together with the deeper tissue (Fig. 6.4a). Now the entire outside of the specimen can be embedded by either placing the two halves into one embedding cassette in the orientation to the patient (Fig. 6.4b). This kind of embedding orientation allows a good orientation (see Fig. 2.7), but it is deviating from the rule and should only be used if the entire tissue can be fitted into one cassette. Following the described embedding rules, i.e., earliest position to the top from right to left, another shape of embedding will result (Fig. 6.4c).

In case of larger scars, the tissue will not fit into one embedding cassette and has to be divided as previously described in Chap. 4. However, in this case it is highly recommendable to follow the previously described embedding rules to avoid confusion.

Large Scar Re-excision After Primary Wound Closure (Exploratory Surgery)

For larger scars it is recommended to first determine the precise localization of expected tumor outgrowths by an exploratory surgery. Here the scar is completely removed for orientation

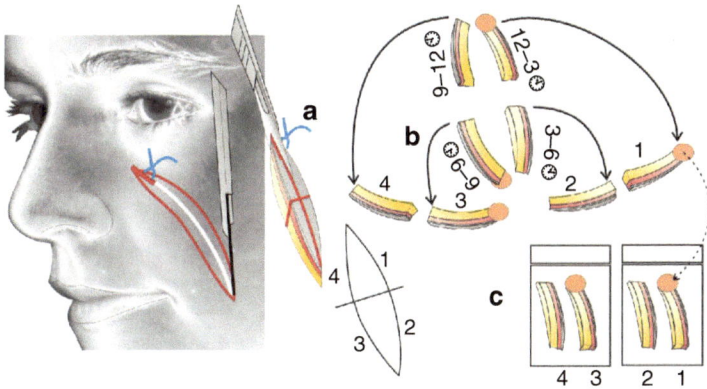

FIGURE 6.5 Large scar re-excision after primary wound closure, embedding clockwise

with a relatively small safety margin and deeper tissue. Then it is divided into smaller pieces fitting into the respective embedding cassettes (Fig. 6.5a red lines). As the entire excised scar will be examined using 3D histology, the pieces should be orientated using clock logic, i.e., in clockwise order (Fig. 6.5b). Now the pieces can be loaded from right to left into the embedding cassette always marking the top of the first strip in each cassette, i.e., the 12 and 6 o'clock (Fig. 6.5c). The embedded scar pieces can now be analyzed for tumor outgrowths and their position relative to the scar can be determined.

The consequent usage of 3D histology in all skin tumor excisions will also allow for a targeted re-excision of tumor outgrowths if the defect was closed with a flap or skin transplantation. Usually such closures shall only be used once the complete removal of the tumor has been injured. However, in some rare cases it might be more efficient to already finally close the defect after the re-excision of small outgrowths concerning one clock time only. Here the risk of a further outgrowth is low. But if in such cases the diagnosis of more tumor-positive tissue will make another re-excision necessary, it can be done after the defect healed completely. The most challenging step in re-excisions after flap closures is the reconstruction in mind of the original defect. Following the topographic changes induced by a flap, the outgrowths can be projected onto the scar and removed with one excision. The re-excision will also allow the possible required correction of the scar from the first surgery.

Chapter 7
Variations for Special Locations and Large, Deep Penetrating Tumors

In this chapter, the excision of tumors growing at special locations such as nose, lips, eyelid, and ear will be discussed. The natural border of the anatomy of these tissues restrains the possibilities for tumor outgrowths and also limits the surgical options to remove the margin. Also, surgery at these locations or the division of the tumor tissue might require special care as the skin can be very thin or very inflexible. Additionally, the excision and division workup of very large tumors which might also penetrate deeper tissues like bones will be described in this chapter in detail. Here particularly, the deep penetration of tumors into other tissues such as bone tissue requires special attention as a full 3D histological workup might not be possible or straightforward. It should be noted that as before, all combinations of excision variations and embedding are freely exchangeable and are only chosen as exemplification. As always, the ultimate goal for all procedures is the full recovery of the entire 3D margin of the tumor specimen for histological evaluation and the following application of these findings onto the respective 3D defect. In this chapter, the plane of the embedded margins and the corresponding histological slide are presented in a simplified margin scheme.

H. Breuninger, P. Adam, *3D Histology Evaluation*
of Dermatologic Surgery, DOI 10.1007/978-1-4471-4438-0_7,
© Springer-Verlag London 2013

Procedures Dealing with Specially Localized Tumors

Some tumor localizations with complex structures will require some variations in excising the tumor specimen. Particularly the nose, lips, eyelids, and ear will require modifications to the previously described procedure. In this chapter, several alternative excision methods for these areas will be described and illustrated. Natural borders such as the ala nasi, the lip, or helix rim are cut in the examples shown here with all layers from outside to inside. The next goal here should also be to save as much tissue as possible in these aesthetically relevant areas. Using 3D histology with its high sensitivity enables high cure rates even if the safety margins are severely reduced.

Removal of a Flat Tumor at the Tip of the Nose

A lot of small tumors do not infiltrate very deeply which is advantageous if located, e.g., at the tip of the nose. To preserve healthy tissue and to allow a nearly scar-free wound healing, the tumor is excised tangentially with a safety margin within the dermis and a slightly deeper cut at the central base position. Prior to this, a punch biopsy of 3–4 mm in the center of the tumor may be advantageous for diagnostic (Fig. 7.1a). For orientation, a marker is set by incision at 12 o'clock

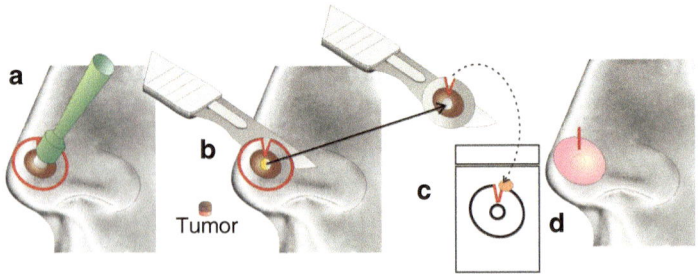

FIGURE 7.1 A flat tumor at the tip of the nose

(Fig. 7.1b). Then the flat tissue is put in a cassette with its outside down in a plane so that it can be used in the histological workup (Fig. 7.1c). The resulting flat defect within the dermis will heal by primary epithelialization (Fig. 2.1d).

A Deep Penetrating Tumor at the Ala Nasi

In regions with natural borders like the ala nasi, 3D histology works as well. In this case, the usual marker is set at 12 o'clock. Then in a first step, the clinical deep infiltrating tumor is excised at its clinical borders together with the nasal entrance rim, cartilage, and parts of the mucosa ala nasi, preserving a thin layer of mucosa (Fig. 7.2a, b). In a second step, a 2–3 mm wide strip is cut off as further safety margin from the border with all layers and parts of the mucosa (Fig. 7.2b), resulting in the shown defect (here the later required re-excisions are also marked). The excised margin tissue is then flattened with its outside down into one plane for embedding. Here additional deep crosswise incisions within the

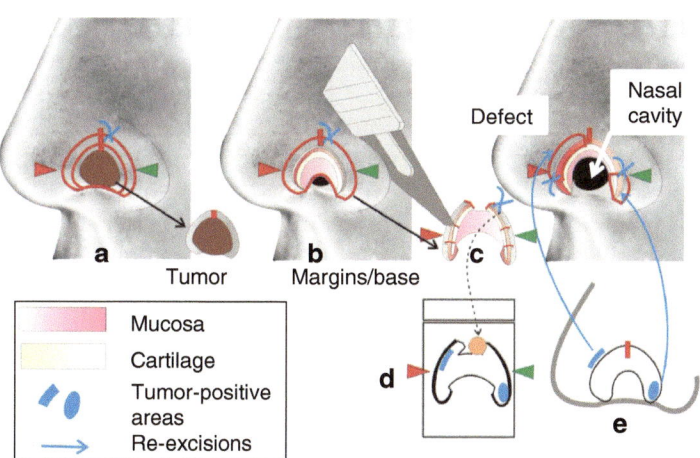

FIGURE 7.2 A deep penetrating tumor at the ala nasi. Handling stiff skin with cartilage by incisions

cartilage of the margin strip might be required (Fig. 7.2c). Figure 7.2d shows the margin scheme with the diagnosed tumor-positive areas (dermal margin 9–11 o'clock and deep at lateral nasal rim). In Figure 7.2e, the corresponding map is seen. Here also the planned re-excisions (skin margin 8–12 o'clock and complete nasal lateral rim) are marked (marker at the earliest clock time) and can then be transferred onto the patient.

A Deep Penetrating Tumor at the Tip of the Nose

Deep penetrating tumors at the tip of the nose require the removal of larger parts of the nose. The excision of this tumor at the tip of the nose follows the same rules as the removal of tumors located at other sites. Also here first, a marker should be placed at the 12 o'clock position, and then the tumor is excised together with a safety margin with the nasal rim and parts of the mucosa ala nasi but saving the important cartilage (Fig. 7.3a). After the excision of the central tumor, unfortunately, outgrowths in the depth between the cartilage parts can be seen clinically. To remove these, the underlying layer of cartilage is marked and cut in a second step, comparable to the excision of the tumor base in other tumors (Fig. 7.3b). For histology, the base is then embedded with its underside facing down (Fig. 7.3d). For a full 3D histology, strips are cut from the border and flattened for embedding with their outside down. Here it is usually necessary to cut the strips several times crosswise as the skin of the nose has a very low flexibility (Fig. 7.3c). Now the entire plane margin can be worked up to histological slides shown schematically in Fig. 7.3d with marked tumor-positive areas (dermal margin 2–4 o'clock and base within the cartilage at tip of the nose). In Figure 7.3e, the corresponding map is seen. Here also the planned re-excisions (skin margin 1–5 o'clock and cartilage at the tip of the nose) are marked (marker at the earliest clock time) and can then be transferred onto the patient.

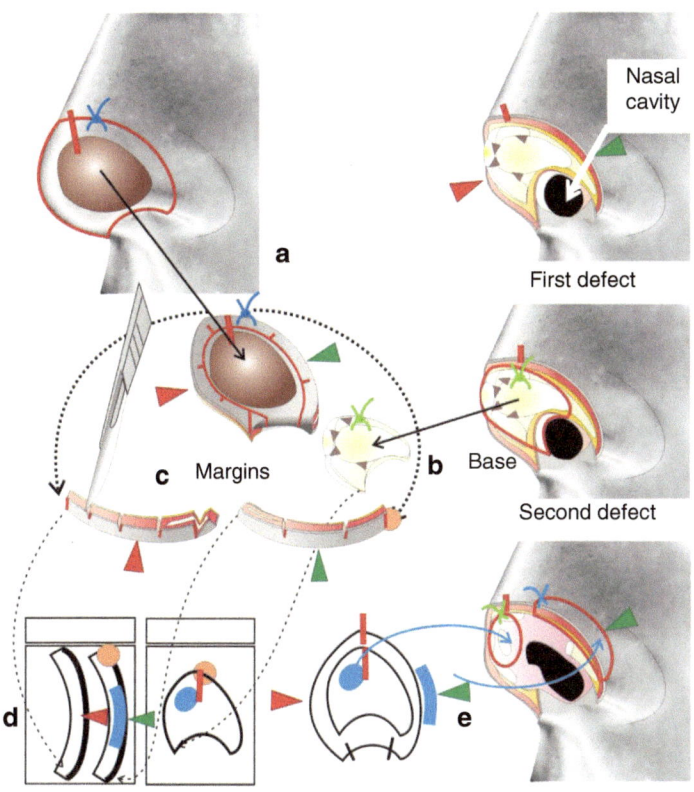

FIGURE 7.3 A deep penetrating tumor at the tip of the nose. Handling stiff skin

Tumors at the Vermillion Border of the Lower Lip

As we have seen in Fig. 7.2, tumors at natural anatomic borders can be excised with all surrounding tissue layers. Like the nose, the lip represents a natural anatomic border. To remove smaller tumors located here, the central tumor is excised with a wedge-shaped excision including a safety margin, the muscle, and parts of the oral mucosa (Fig. 7.4a). For histology, 2–3 mm wide strips are cut from the borders of the

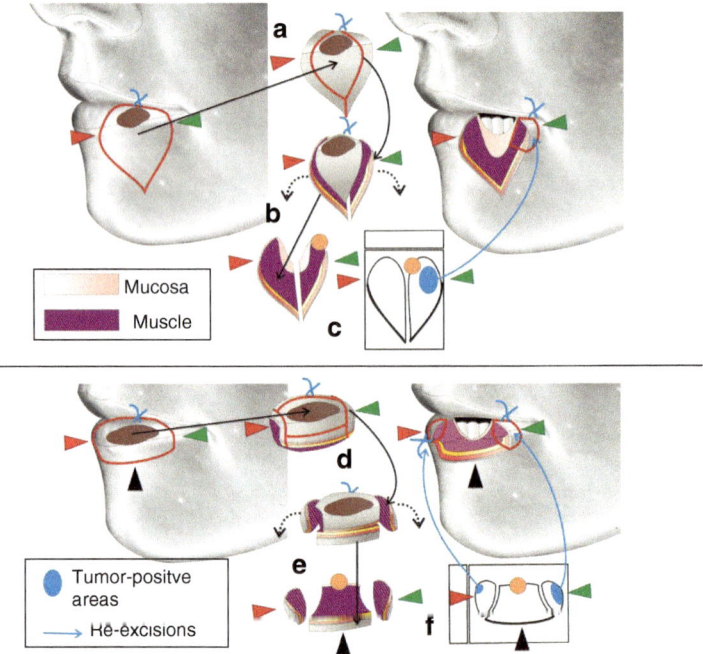

<figure>

Mucosa

Muscle

Tumor-positve areas

Re-excisions
</figure>

FIGURE 7.4 Tumors at the vermillion border of the lower lip. Wedge or boxlike excision

wedge representing the entire 3D margin (Fig. 7.4b) and leaving the central tumor material behind. An excision of the base section is not necessary due to the natural anatomic border. The margin strips are pressed flat with their outside down in a plane representing the complete outside of the tumor specimen. After histology, tumor outgrowths can be diagnosed and respective re-excisions planned (Fig. 7.4c), here 3 o'clock at the vermillion border.

Larger tumors in this area should be excised using a box-shaped excision. Here the tumor is excised with a safety margin together with the muscle and parts of the oral mucosa in one piece (Fig. 7.4d). From this box, the borders are cut off as demonstrated before in the square procedure, and the central tumor material is removed above the base (Fig. 7.4e). Strips are pressed flat with their outside down in a plane and be processed in the histological workup. The 12 o'clock position was changed from the top of the cassette to its side to fill it most efficiently. In the scheme shown here, the tumor presents tumor-positive areas at the vermillion border medial (9 o'clock) with a smaller part and lateral (3 o'clock) with a larger part within the muscle (Fig. 7.4f). Now the required re-excisions can be planned.

Tumors at the Eyelid

Small tumors at the eyelid canthus can be excised with the help of a needle. Then the surrounding tissue is cut out with the cartilage muscle and parts of the conjunctiva of the lid border using a little hook to grab the tissue (Fig. 7.5a). To prepare this excised tissue bowl for embedding, it can simply be cut in the middle and folded open so that it can be pressed flat with the outside facing down (Fig. 7.5b). Now the specimen will represent the whole margin and the base of the specimen. Here the tumor presents an outgrowth at the dermal margin (5–7 o'clock) and requires a re-excision of the lid skin 4–8 o'clock as indicated (marker at the earliest clock time) (Fig. 7.5c).

Tumors growing on the thin skin of the lower lid should be excised in two steps. First, the central tumor is excised very thinly only down to the subcutaneous tissue (Fig. 7.5d). Then the lateral safety margin and the deeper central tissue, i.e., superficial part of the periorbital muscle, which is located here very superficial, are removed together. The preparation for histology follows as usual in cutting a strip of the border and leaving the central base in one piece (Fig. 7.5e). Now these parts of tissue can be histologically worked up. In the case shown here, the tumor represents outgrowths which are shown here on the margin scheme (dermal margin 3–1 (3–14) o'clock and base 8–10 o'clock) (Fig. 7.5f) and the map which should have been created for documentation (Fig. 7.5g). These findings result in the necessary indicated re-excision of

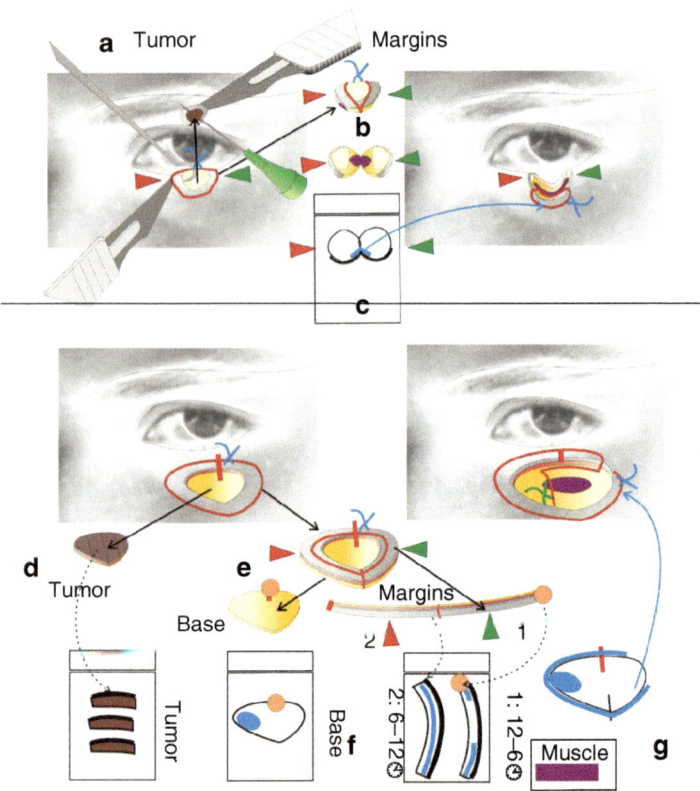

FIGURE 7.5 Tumors at the eyelid. Handling thin skin: first flat tumor excision then margins and base

the skin margins from 3 to 2 (2–14) o'clock with a marker at 2 o'clock and at the base 7–11 o'clock, respectively.

Tumors at the Helix

The removal of tumors at the helix is similar to the removal of larger tumors at the lip (Fig. 7.4d–f). Also here, the tumor is excised together with a safety margin, the cartilage, and helix backside in a box-shaped specimen. Therefore, the borders will have a square shape and can be cut off as

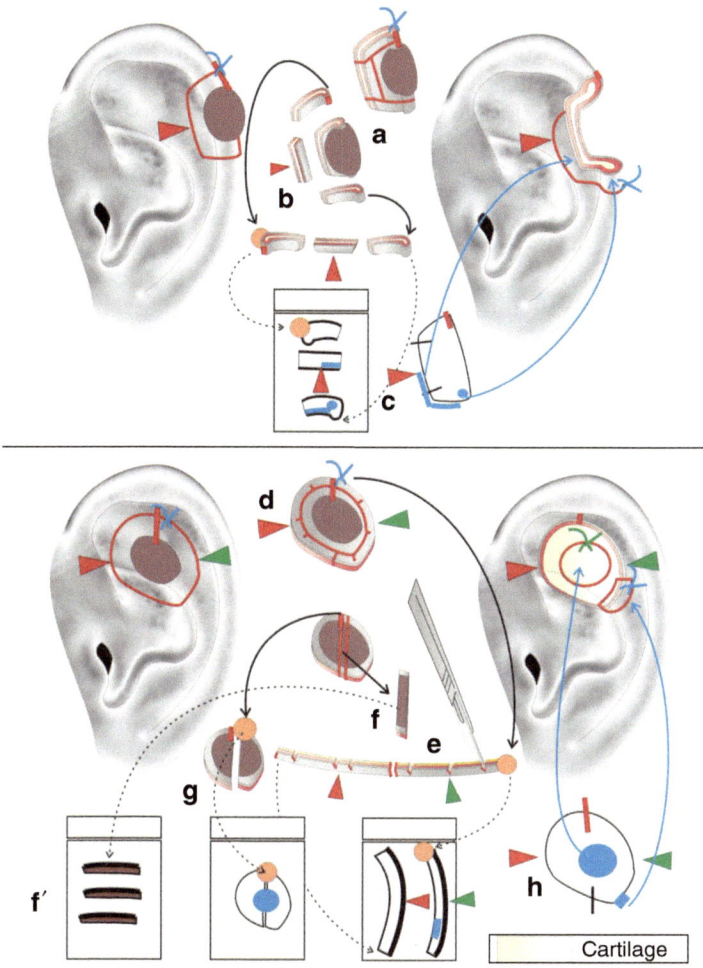

FIGURE 7.6 Tumors at the helix. Tumors at different areas with different degrees of infiltration to the depth

shown in the square procedure or in the demonstrated case of the lip, representing front and backside of the helix rim. Here the margins will be marked for topographic orientation at 12 o'clock only to avoid a mix-up (Fig. 7.6b).

However, close attention should be paid to the inside–outside orientation of the strip. They are put within the cassette resulting in a histological slide shown in the margin scheme (Fig. 7.6c). In the case shown here, the tumor presents outgrowths at the dermal margin 6–9 o'clock and within the cartilage at 6 o'clock (helix rim). This requires the indicated re-excision (complete helix rim 6 o'clock and skin margin 6–10 o'clock with a marker at 6 o'clock).

The skin at the concha helix is extremely thin, and it is therefore difficult to excise tumor and safety margin in independent steps. To remove tumors in this area, the excision should be done in one step removing the tumor with safety margin at the side and depth down to the perichondrium together (Fig. 7.6d). For histology, the side margins are then cut from the border of the excised specimen. To press their outside down, it might be helpful to use incisions to flatten these parts (Fig. 7.6e). As the skin of the ear has a very low flexibility and is very thin, the removal of the base is usually impossible. Therefore, it is recommendable to cut only a very small middle section of the tumor (alternatively, a punch biopsy can be taken) for diagnostic (Fig. 7.6f, f′) and use the remaining parts of the tissue for the base (Fig. 7.6g). Now the complete margins and base can be investigated. In this case, the tumor presents dermal positive areas 4–5 o'clock and at the base central as shown on the map used for documentation (Fig. 7.6h). Further re-excisions will remove the central cartilage and skin 4–6 o'clock marked at 4 o'clock.

Taken together, the examples shown here so far indicate the large variations of excision methods for tumors grown at special areas. If complex structures in the head and neck region are infiltrated, the 3D histologic procedure has to be adapted to the natural borders. Drawings or photographs of the topographic situation may be suitable to use for topographic orientation rather than the mere description of the histological finding.

Treatment of Larger Tumors with Penetrations into Deeper Tissues

The treatment of larger tumors with outgrowths penetrating deeper tissues such as the bone requires also special attention in their excision and division. Particularly, tumor infiltrations into the bone will have to be removed in parts using a chisel. As bone structures impair the histological evaluation, these parts have to be decalcified separately before they can be embedded. Only then the histological evaluation using H&E staining can be realized. In cases where tumor borders are unclear or the tumors are large and have deeply reaching infiltrations, excisions in multiple steps will be necessary. The following section will focus on the special requirements in the treatment of these tumors.

Tumor at the Forehead with Infiltration of the Bone

Larger tumors at the forehead are likely to develop infiltrations in the bone underneath. For the excision, the tumor is first removed with safety margin including the muscle but leaving the periosteum in situ if it is clinically not infiltrated (Fig. 7.7a). Here the tumor-positive areas are marked on the margin scheme and on the map which is used for documentation (Fig. 7.7b). The example shown here presents positive dermal margins at 12–4 with a little gap at 2 o'clock, 7–8, and 11 o'clock. Furthermore, a positive outgrowth at the central base is diagnosed.

For the required re-excision in this case, the entire margin 10–5 (10–17) o'clock is removed in one excision, marked at 10 o'clock and the area 6–9 o'clock separately (Fig. 7.7c). At the base, now the periosteum is removed using either a raspatorium or a chisel (Fig. 7.7c). Due to the widespread infiltration shown in this example, a second re-excision will be required,

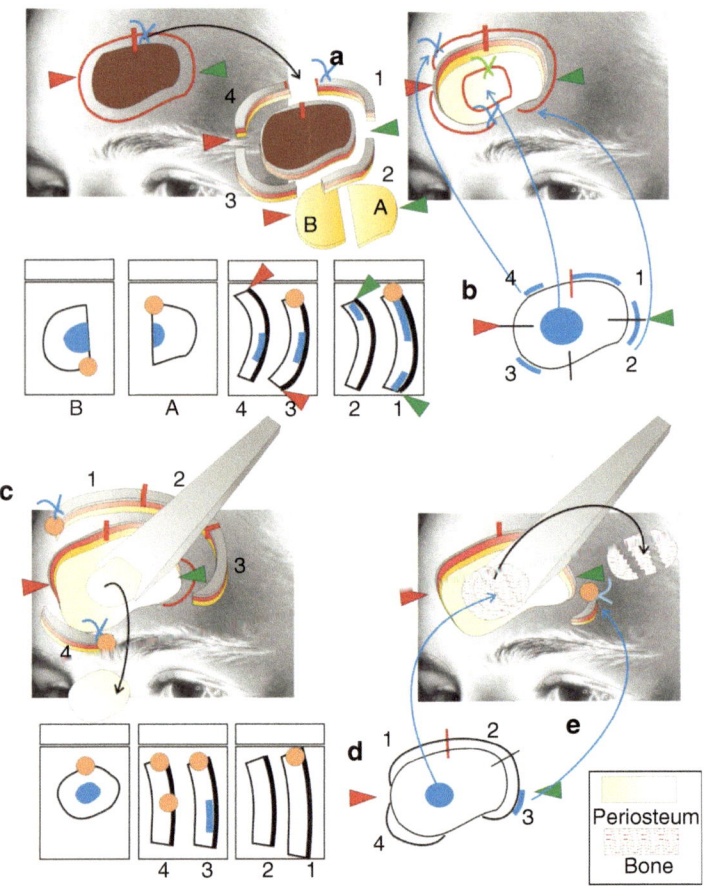

FIGURE 7.7 A tumor at the front of the head infiltrating the bone. The areas of histological detected tumor outgrowths are re-excised

as 3D histology of the first re-excision still shows positive areas at the dermal margin 3–4 o'clock and the periosteum as indicated here on the margin scheme or map (Fig. 7.7d). Therefore, a second re-excision at the margin and a deeper layer of the bone are necessary (Fig. 7.7e). Note that due to the brittle properties of the bone, this tissue cannot be removed in one piece, and the material has to be saved in parts. As mentioned before, bone will impair the histology.

Therefore, it will be necessary to demineralize these tissue parts before they can be processed normally. After the second re-excision, margins were tumor-free.

Tumor Infiltrating Complex Structures of the Nose and Lip: First Step

In order to preserve as much healthy tissue as possible, larger tumors in complex and aesthetically relevant areas have to be removed carefully and in several steps. Depending on the location, the safety margins can be adjusted to the size of the tumor and the aesthetic importance of the surrounding structures. This is necessary to preserve as much tissue as possible in each of the surgeries. Therefore, the first surgery should excise the tumor only with a moderate safety margin of 2–3 mm of normal-looking skin. In the depth, only a minimal required amount of muscle tissue should be used to save the mimic muscles as it looks clinically normal (Fig. 7.8a and defect).

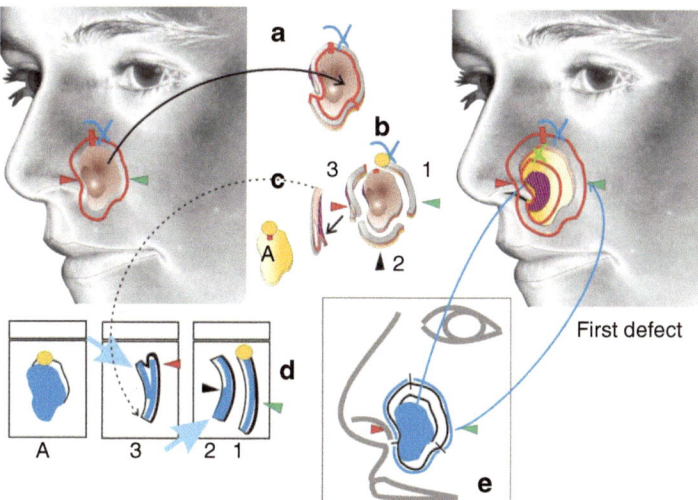

FIGURE 7.8 A tumor infiltrating complex structures of the nose and lip: first step (lateral ala nasi and parts of the cheek in the depth with parts of the muscles)

From the isolated tumor, the safety margins are divided (Fig. 7.8b). The here also isolated complex ala nasi is part of the outer margin as well and here part of the third margin section (Fig. 7.8c). In this case, separate cassettes for the ala nasi and base are required, resulting in the respective histological slides shown here (Fig. 7.8d). Such structures also provide the pathologist a further orientation point and therefore allow a better orientation in the histological evaluation. Due to the relative complexity of tumors like the one shown here, a drawing or photo would be highly desirable to aid in orientation. Here the tumor presents positive outgrowths in all directions, concerning the dermal margin 12–12, deep margin until the lower border at ala nasi and upper lip (blue arrows), and in a large area of the base, especially towards the nose making another re-excision necessary, which can now be planned as shown (Fig. 7.8e).

Tumor Infiltrating Complex Structures of the Nose and Lip: Second Step

In the first re-excision, additional 4 mm of the complete margin is now removed. The now larger margin is then divided into 4 parts. While part 4 is ending at its border at the ala nasi where all layers have been cut, part 3 ends in the depth of the nose entrance (Fig. 7.9a little black arrows). At the base, deep muscle structures are removed until the periosteum of the upper jaw and the mucosa of the upper lip (Fig. 7.9b). Clinically, both of these tissues appear not to be infiltrated. Also in this step, the standard division and marking rules for embedding can be applied leading to histological sections shown here (Fig. 7.9c). Now the tumor margins present also areas which are not infested. Tumor-positive areas are to find at dermal margin 2–4, 7–8, and 11–1 (11–13) o'clock dermal and deeper layers and base until periosteum and mucosa. This allows a targeted planning of the next re-excision (Fig. 7.9d).

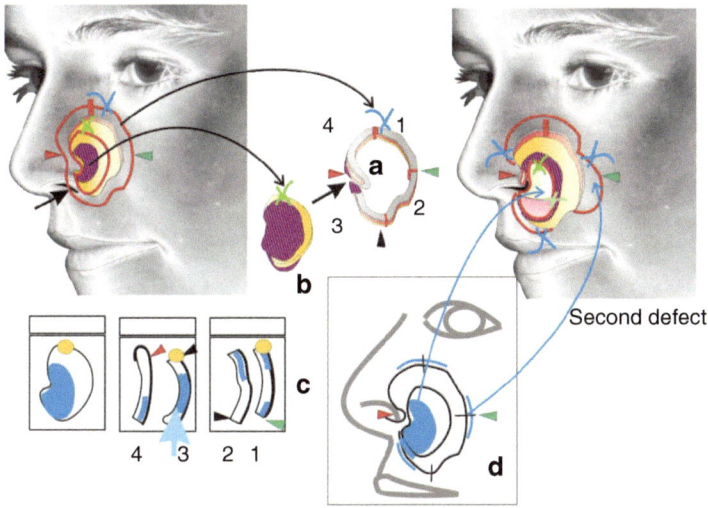

FIGURE 7.9 A tumor infiltrating complex structures of the nose and lip: second step (complete margin and depth until mucosa and periosteum)

Tumor Infiltrating Complex Structures of the Nose and Lip: Third and Fourth Step

At the cheek, the margins are now excised with a larger 6 mm wide excision (Fig. 7.10a, b) to minimize the number of re-excisions. From these excised margins, a smaller 2–3 mm strip from the outside has to be isolated for 3D histology in order to enable embedding (Fig. 7.10a′, b′). It is therefore possible to re-excise also larger parts of the margin, if the smaller strip of the outer margin required for embedding is cut off separately. Due to the more sensitive area of the lip, the re-excision in this area should still only isolate as little tissue as necessary. Therefore, only a margin of 3 mm skin and muscle is isolated (Fig. 7.10c). This smaller strip can then be embedded directly showing the skin and underlying muscle. At the

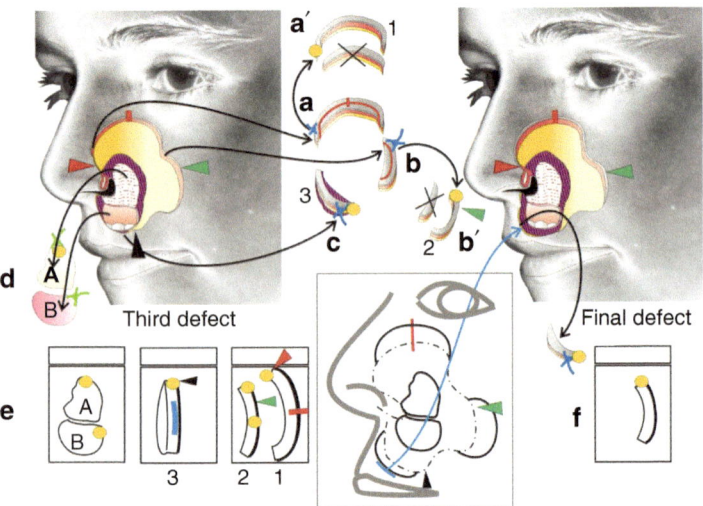

FIGURE 7.10 A tumor infiltrating complex structures of the nose and lip: third and fourth step (tumor-positive parts of the margin and in the depth with periosteum and mucosa)

base of the tumor, the periosteum of the upper jaw and the mucosa of the upper lip are excised in two parts A and B leaving the bone and teeth with gingiva (Fig. 7.10d). All these isolated margin strips are to be embedded resulting in the representative histological slides as shown in the margin scheme. The second strip in the first cassette is independent from the first; therefore, both got a marker at the earliest clock time. To avoid confusion, the second strip gets a second marker (Fig. 7.10e). After this third re-excision, the only tumor-positive areas can be found in the dermal upper lip section (7–8 o'clock on the map). After the now fourth re-excision of the upper lip, the tissue is healthy (Fig. 7.10f), and the defect can be closed.

Such multi-step procedures have the advantage that much more healthy tissue can be preserved, which in the case to the face or other sensitive areas will greatly improve the development of smaller scars.

So far only examples in the face were described. All of the described example procedures can be transferred to other areas of the body. However, with increasing tumor size at the other parts of the body, the procedure requires special attention. Here the area is often much larger and the subcutaneous tissue much thicker. Nevertheless, it is possible to achieve a relatively efficient full histological workup if the simple embedding rules are followed. If the fatty tissue parts are isolated, only one strip should be put in one cassette making the marking of margin tissue sections unnecessary. Then only the parts of the base have to be marked following the clock logic. In the following, an example of such a large tumor at the upper arm and shoulder will be discussed.

Large Tumor at the Lateral Upper Arm and Shoulder: First Step

The first initial tumor excision is performed with a safety margin of 10 mm at the sides and down to the muscle at the central areas (Fig. 7.11a) resulting in the shown defect with a muscle layer in the center. The tumor specimen is then divided as described previously in margin and base in which muscle is visible (Fig. 7.11b). The separated margin is flattened, as always with the outside facing down, and will be divided in this case in eight parts and placed in embedding cassettes in a clockwise order from left to right (here only one strip per cassette due to the thickness of the tissue). Similarly, the base is cut in four parts with markers for orientation at the lowest clock time (Fig. 7.11c). After embedding, the histological sectioning will result in the representative slides shown here (Fig. 7.11d). After the histological evaluation of all the slides, a tumor map with marked tumor-positive areas can be drawn for documentation: tumor-positive areas dermal and subdermal 4–7, 10, and 11 o'clock and base of central 5–7 o'clock (Fig. 7.11e),

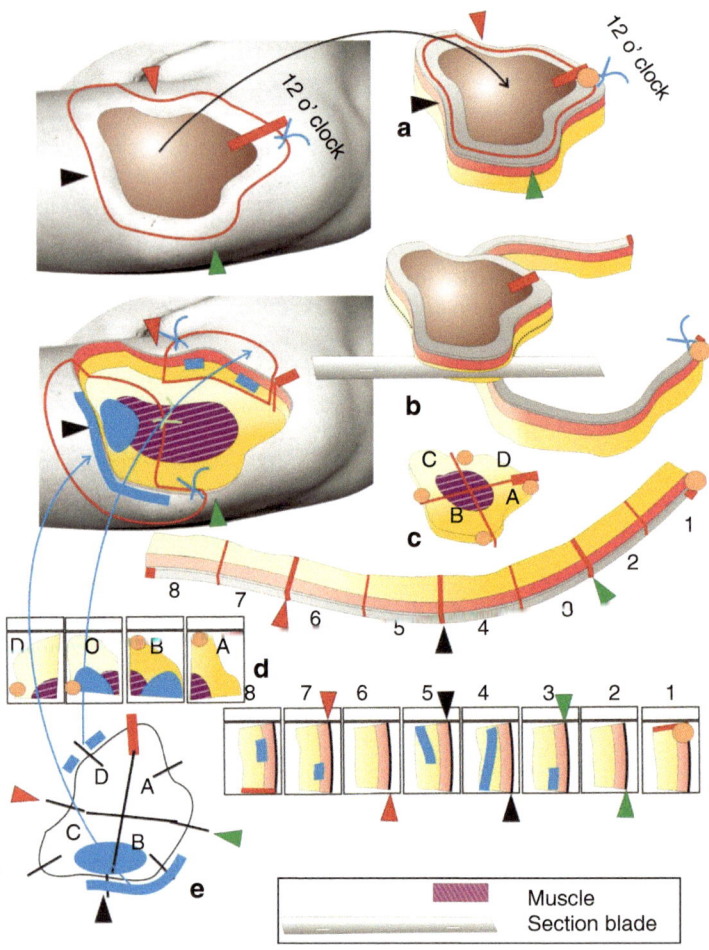

FIGURE 7.11 A large tumor at the lateral upper left arm – shoulder (12 o'clock), first step with tumor-positive areas at the margins and base

allowing the surgeon to plan the next re-excision (shown on the defect as red lines together with the topographical markers).

Large Tumor at the Lateral Upper Arm and Shoulder: Second Step

Also the re-excision is done with a safety margin of another 10 mm and down to the muscle in the center. Due to the broadness of the re-excised margins, a smaller 4 mm strip of the outer margin has to be isolated as described before (Fig. 7.12a). Again the margin parts are embedded in individual cassettes resulting in the representative sections as shown here (Fig. 7.12b). The histological evaluation in this case presents only a small dermal tumor-positive area in the subdermal layer around the 5 o'clock position (see map in Fig. 7.12c or slide 2 in Fig. 7.12b), which can be removed in one further re-excision as indicated in the defect (red lines).

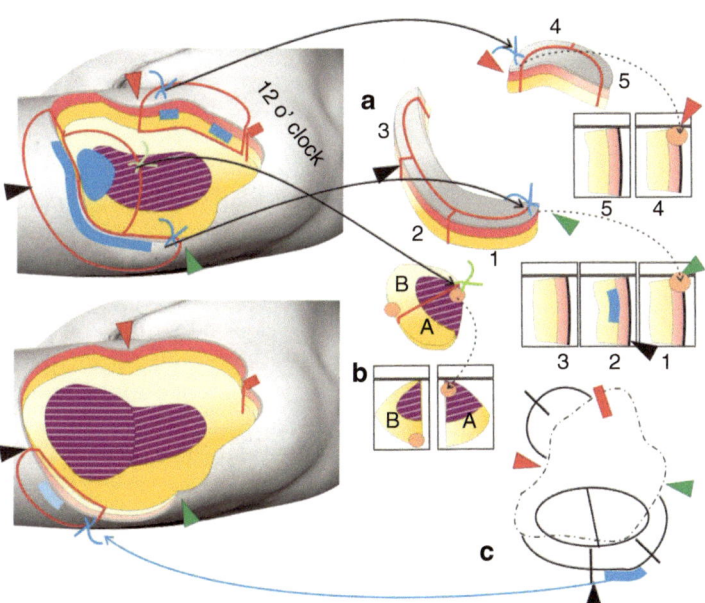

FIGURE 7.12 A large tumor at the lateral upper left arm – shoulder – second step with a positive margin at 5 o'clock

In case of tumors in the deeper soft tissue like liposarco-mas or similar entities, 3D histology can be used as well to ensure the full removal of the tumor until clear margins are ensured. Even very small infiltrations of less than 1 mm can be detected. However, these tumors are surrounded by the soft tissues, and hence the procedure has to be modified. In these cases, two markers are necessary for topographic ori-entation: 1 at 12 o'clock and the other at the point of the skin surface. If the tumor is larger, a formalin fixation before the tissue division is usually advantageous as the tis-sue becomes more rigid. Then it is recommendable to first divide the tumor specimen horizontally. After that, a mar-gin border of approximately 4 mm thickness is cut off and divided in parts fitting in a cassette. Rigid fixed tissue can be pressed into a plane after embedding in wax as is was described earlier in Fig. 3.6. Unlike in the conventional technique, here the entire 3D margins of the tumor can be investigated to ensure clear margins and therefore the full removal of the tumor.

Subcutaneous Tumor at the Chest

In tumors growing in deeper soft tissue, the size can only be estimated. Therefore, the primary tumor excision has to be done with a sufficient amount of surrounding tissue. In this example shown here, the excision was done with a small part of the skin and safety margin to all sides. In the depth, muscle tissue was included resulting in a specimen of about 60 mm in diameter resulting in an orange-shaped specimen. Now two markers are necessary: 1 at 12 o'clock position relative to the top of the head and one at the ventral, i.e., lower surface (Fig. 7.13a). The tumor specimen is then divided at the ventral marker in a ventral and dorsal part (Fig. 7.13b). This may be easier if the specimen is fixed in formalin as the tissue will be more rigid. From the outside of both (ventral and dorsal) parts, the margins of approx. 4 mm thickness can be cut off like the peeling of an orange. Now markers are set at the edge representing the earliest clock time and processed as usual

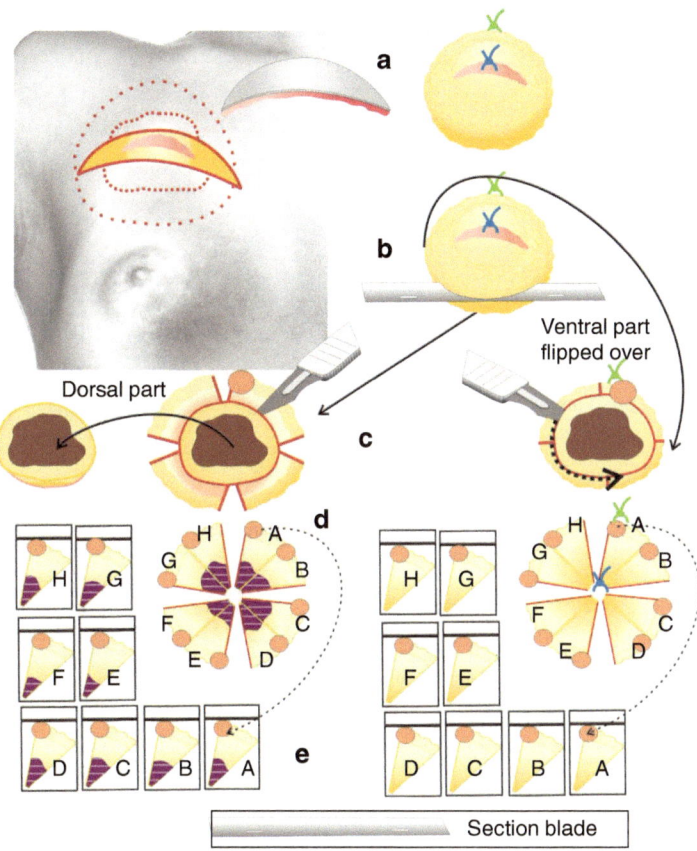

FIGURE 7.13 A subcutaneous tumor at the chest. Cutting off the 3D outside

(Fig. 7.13d). The left middle tumor parts are put aside for further investigation (Fig. 7.13c). The margins of each side can then be flattened by cutting them into pieces fitting in the cassettes. In the case shown here, this will result in eight pieces of ventral part and another eight pieces of dorsal part. As always, each piece should be embedded with the outside facing down. If this procedure is followed, the resulting cassettes will represent the entire 3D margin outside the tumor which can then be evaluated histologically (Fig. 7.13e).

Chapter 8
How to Perform 3D Histology on Different Types of Tumors

General Rules for 3D Histology

3D histology is intended for tumors at difficult sites where a tissue-saving surgical technique is needed or if local R0 resection must be ensured due to the aggressive growth of the tumor (Table 8.1) [1]. Precondition for this technique is a continuous local, clinically invisible infiltration of the tumor. Therefore, the margins of the excised tumor have to be investigated histologically in order to verify total removal of the tumor. For safety reasons, it is recommendable to increase the width of the safety margins in the primary excision of the tumor relative to the overall size of the tumor. Only in more distinguished locations with important structures or for aesthetical reasons, it is recommendable to choose smaller safety margins in order to save healthy tissue. However, it is imperative that in any case, the full removal is diagnosed by the presence of histologically clear margins.

Margin Widths for the First Excision

All malignant tumors of the skin and some in situ local tumors (M. Paget or M. Bowen) show irregular, often asymmetric, mainly horizontal subclinical infiltrations with a lateral extent

H. Breuninger, P. Adam, *3D Histology Evaluation of Dermatologic Surgery*, DOI 10.1007/978-1-4471-4438-0_8, © Springer-Verlag London 2013

TABLE 8.1 Tumor types suitable for 3D histology

1. Basal cell carcinoma, especially infiltrative types

2. Squamous cell carcinomas that have infiltrated the subcutaneous layer or have moderate to poor differentiation. Desmoplastic type without or with perineural infiltration

3. Lentigo maligna, lentigo maligna melanoma, acral lentiginous melanoma, desmoplastic melanoma

4. Dermatofibrosarcoma protuberans

5. Merkel cell carcinoma

6. Extramammary Paget's disease perianal and genital Bowen disease

7. Recurrent tumors

8. Experimental: very rare soft tissue sarcomas

of zero to several centimeters [2–6]. When in-depth infiltrations are present, they are often asymmetric as well and hard to predict. However, tumor infiltrations into the depth usually are limited to the subcutaneous layer or mimic muscles. On the other hand deep infiltrations into skeletal muscle cartilage and bone are not uncommon. Deep, destructive and larger infiltrations may be visible preoperatively to a certain degree on a CT or MRT scan, but neither technology will allow a prediction of the infiltrations down to a histological level. In all cases complete excision requires a good knowledge of local patterns of infiltration of various types of skin tumors.

Excisions may be performed singly or in series ("staged surgical excision"). Immediate closure of the wound is possible, especially if the excision was done with wide margins (see Fig. 8.1 for basal cell carcinomas) and the closure does not interfere with precise topographic orientation of any potentially necessary re-excisions. Alternatively, a temporary protective bandage may be used until the histological results become available. Once tumor-free margins have been achieved, final closure of the defect is performed with plastic reconstruction or via secondary healing.

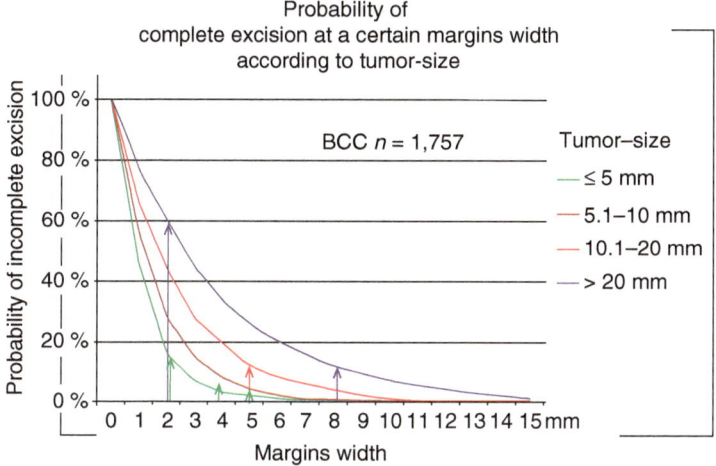

FIGURE 8.1 Rate of tumor-positive margins depending on margin width

TABLE 8.2 Premises for the estimation of the margin width

Two primary premises:

1. Location: e.g., *small* at the nose, eyelids, lip, ear, and fingers; middle at forehead, cheek, chin, and neck; large at the trunk and proximal extremities

2. Method of histological examination. *Larger* if the examination has gaps, *smaller* with 3D histology

Two secondary premises:

1. Tumor size: *smaller* in small tumors, *larger* in large tumors

2. Tumor type: *smaller* in solid types, *larger* in infiltrating types

Basal Cell Carcinoma (BCC)

Basal cell carcinoma is the most common malignant skin tumor. For the complete excision of these types of tumors, the margin width can be chosen individually from 1 mm up to 20 mm and is mainly determined by (1) the tumor type and size, (2) the location, and (3) method of histological examination (Table 8.2).

There is a direct relationship between the tumor diameter and the width of the infiltration, but this relationship is again depending on the localization and is therefore relative.

The figure shows the rates for different tumor diameters. The larger the tumor, the higher is the rate of positive margins. The larger the margin width, the lower is the rate of positive margins)

In difficult or sensitive locations, e.g., nose, eyelids, or ear, it is desirable to save normal tissue. However, the smaller the margin, the higher will be the rate of required re-excisions. If the margin width of primary excision was 2 mm, the probability of incomplete eradication for small tumors >5 mm diameter is only 16 % but raises up to 59 % for large tumors >20 mm in diameter. Often these re-excisions do not affect the entire margin, and therefore if followed histologically, healthy tissue can be saved, and the final defect will be smaller, adapted to the real tumor extension. If the safety margin width is increased to 5 mm for small tumors of 5 mm, the eradication rate drops even further to 2 %. Also for larger tumors a wider safety margin will decrease the rates for required re-excisions substantially like for tumors up to 20 mm diameter excised with 5 mm margin. Here the first excision only is incomplete in 12 % of the cases. Larger tumors of more than 20 mm have to be excised with a primary safety margin of 8 mm to reach rates of only 12 % unclear or tumor-positive margins.

Particularly in larger tumors the histological workup should be performed using a method without gaps (see Chap. 9) and a higher sensitivity to detect tumor infiltrations, like the here described 3D histology. To avoid too many re-excisions, the margin width can be adjusted in a tumor versus location adaptation, i.e., can be more generous in regions where a larger defect will not complicate the defect closure. Also, if tumor-positive margins have been found in the primary excision, the re-excision margins of the following steps should be adapted to the extension of the tumor in the margins and to the location as well. It should be noted that the cure rates for BCCs using 3D histology with paraffin sections can be up to 99 % [7, 8].

Squamous Cell Carcinoma (SCC)

SCC has a similar lateral subclinical infiltration like the BCC, but in depth the infiltration reaches much deeper. Here the deep subcutaneous layer, fascia, muscle, cartilage, or periosteum are much more frequently infiltrated than in BCCs. However, also here a tumor versus location adapted primary excision as described above for BCC can be done. Also here paraffin sections are recommended as in cryo-sections small outgrowths can be easily overseen. Following all of these precautions, cure rates of common SCC can reach up to 97 % [7, 9, 10].

The desmoplastic type of SCC with or without perineural and perivascular infiltration often has tremendous subclinical infiltrations, which sometimes need numerous surgeries to be entirely removed. Even with 3D histology using paraffin section, the local recurrence rate is 24 % [3, 5, 9] indicating that the fine infiltrating strands of one cell layer cannot be detected by microscopy using conventional stains such as H&E. Here immunostaining with CK 5/CK 14 seems to be helpful but also not complete. Therefore, the excision of an additional margin of 5–10 mm after R0-resection and/or a postoperative radiation is recommended.

Extramammary Paget's Disease, Bowen's Disease

Tumors of this kind show an exclusive horizontal spread without deep infiltration especially in the perianal and perigenital region. As for BCCs and SCCs, the surgical approach is a tumor versus location adapted primary excision. Especially Paget's disease can have an exorbitant subclinical extent often sometimes several centimeters (Fig. 8.2) or even up to 10 cm. Therefore, a primary excision margin of 10 mm is recommended [6, 11]. Nevertheless, local cure rates of extramammary Paget's disease are relatively low (75 %) despite using 3D histology with paraffin sections. Here immunostaining with C7 can be useful to detect tumor-positive cells in the margin. It is important to say that a base control in the 3D histological workup is not necessary due to the superficial growth.

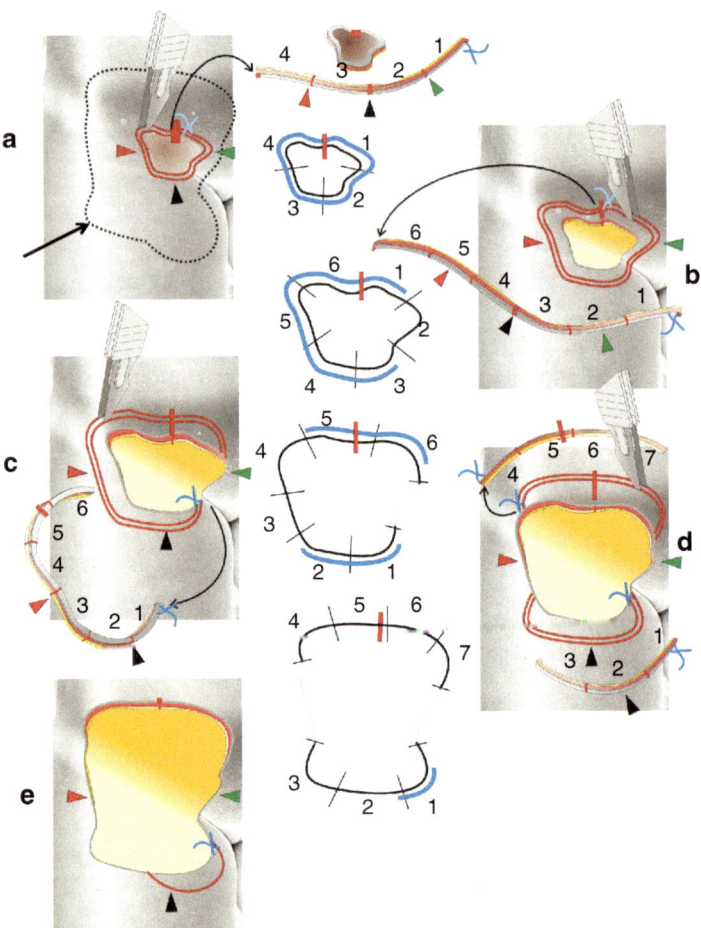

FIGURE 8.2 Paget's disease at a groin, multiple re-excisions at the margins

Paget's Disease at the Groin

Since this type of tumor often has an unclear border, the end of the tumor has to be determined in surgery using 3D histology. In a first operation a margin rim in 10 mm distance to the visible border of the tumor is cut off with a double scalpel. After that the tumor part can be excised. The recovered safety margin is then divided into several pieces, here 4, fitting in embedding cassettes (Fig. 8.2a, see numbering). As mentioned before, this type of tumors only grows superficially; therefore, the base usually does not have to be investigated.

The histological evaluation of the margin strips showed that the 10 mm safety margin was fully infested with tumor tissue, making further exploratory surgeries necessary. In several in about 10 mm steps each time taken, a margin strip is recovered with a double scalpel, divided and histologically investigated until the entire margin is clear (Fig. 8.2b–e). Thick black lines on the maps indicate the explored excision lines; blue markers indicate tumor-infested tissue being diagnosed. These rather generous margin explorations are necessary due to the exclusive widespread subclinical growth of this disease and to avoid too many excision steps. The remaining tissue between the excised strip and the defect has to be removed. The resulting defect can heal secondarily very well in most of the affected localizations (groin, perigenital, and perianal). In very sensible areas resection margins can be taken smaller, and a higher number of exploratory steps, but more targeted and therefore less invasive, might be required.

Lentigo Maligna, Lentigo Maligna Melanoma, Acral Lentiginous Melanoma, and Desmoplastic Melanoma

These melanocytic tumor entities show a mostly exclusive horizontal continuous spread. This is in contrast to other entities of melanoma such as superficial spreading or nodular melanoma which show a discontinuous spread [12]. Only the tumor entity of the desmoplastic melanoma type is infiltrating deep layers. The excision of these types of tumors follows again a tumor versus location adapted primary excision with a safety margin. While for all lentiginous types with a superficial growing the lateral safety margins have to be analyzed using 3D histology, the desmoplastic requires also the analysis of the base.

For lentiginous types of melanoma, such a tissue-saving approach has the same healing rates than surgery with a large margin width of 20 mm [5,13–16]. Lentigo maligna melanoma on the face can be treated with a small excision margin analyzing the dermis only and leaving the subcutaneous tissue in situ. Hence, the defect will be very superficial, and important structures can be saved. At locations where skin grafts are resulting in good wound closure, the resulting defects can easily be closed using such grafts without leaving a dent at the scar. This superficial excision will be explained for some special localizations in the next figure (Fig. 8.3). As for Paget's disease a base control in these exclusively superficially growing tumors is not necessary.

Lentigo Maligna Melanoma

Tumors of this type can primary be excised with a safety margin of 2–5 mm leaving subcutaneous tissue of the patient. For the full histological workup, strips are cut from the borders of the excision and processed as described (Fig. 8.3a, b with the resulting histological slides).

In the next example shown here at the helix rim, the tumor is excised as before with a safety margin and the complete dermis only leaving cartilage in situ. Strips are cut from the borders and processed as described (Fig. 8.3c, d showing the resulting histological slides). The resulting defect can be covered by a skin transplantation as the cartilage with its perichondrium was saved.

Acral lentiginous melanoma can be treated with a location adapted primary excision with view millimeters, avoiding overtreatment, e.g., amputations. A control of the base especially at the distal acres is necessary because sometimes deeper infiltrations occur due to the often late diagnosis of these melanomas. With 3D histology the local cure rate is high (98 %); however, in some cases immunostaining with melan A is helpful [5].

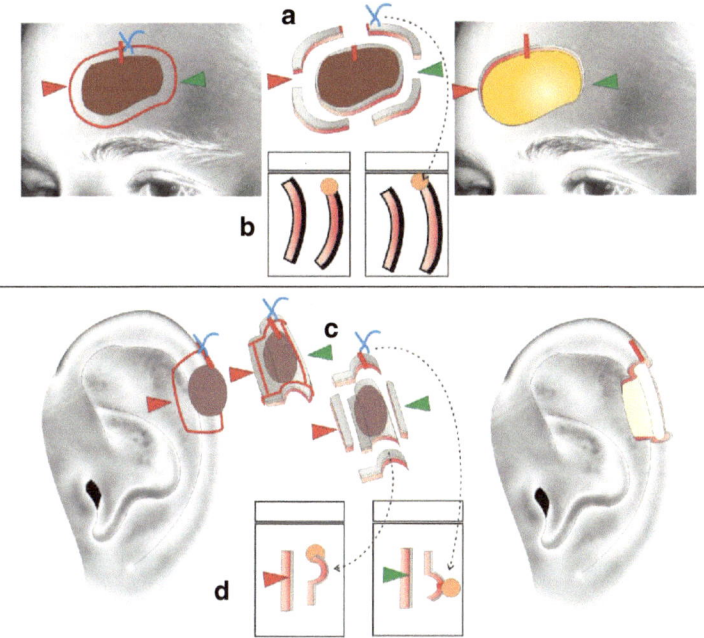

FIGURE 8.3 Lentigo maligna melanoma. Excision with dermis only

Acral Lentiginous Melanoma

In this case acral melanomas at the big toe at the nail matrix and heal are illustrated. The tumor is excised with a safety margin of less than 5 mm in normal skin (Fig. 8.4d) but always with the complete anatomic unit of the nail apparatus. As this tumor is infiltrating deeper tissues, the central tissue should be excised down to the bone. In the shown case the central tumor is excised in one step together with the lateral margins. After that the base with periosteum and a small layer of the bone is removed (Fig. 8.4a). For the histological workup strips are cut from the borders and processed as described. In the shown case here, tumor-positive areas (in situ acral melanoma) were found at 12–1 and 5–6 o'clock. Therefore, a re-excision in these areas has to be done (Fig. 8.4b) until only healthy tissue

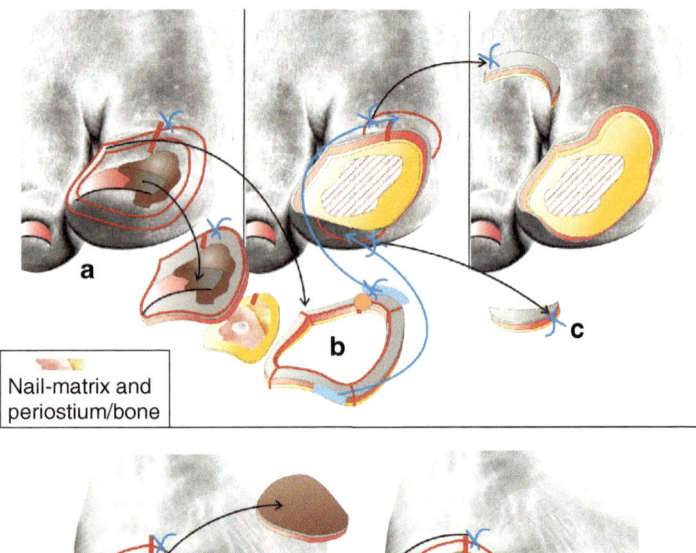

Nail-matrix and
periostium/bone

FIGURE 8.4 Acral lentiginous melanoma

is recovered. A two-step excision of an acral lentiginous melanoma at the heel is shown (Fig. 8.4c). By the way the defect
can heal by secondary intention with excellent results.

Dermatofibrosarcoma Protuberans (DFSP)

DFSP sometimes have a continuous infiltration of a considerable size. Infiltrations of several cm in mainly horizontal
direction within the dermis or subcutaneous layer up to 7 cm
are found [4]. However, also deeper tissues down to fascia
and muscle can be infested. The margin width of primary
excision can be tumor versus location adapted with 5–10 mm.
An example of 3D histology controlled surgery of a DFSP on

the left upper arm is shown in Figs. 7.11 and 7.12. For these tumors, tumor infiltrations can usually be seen in H&E-stained slides. Only in special cases CD-34 immunostaining might be required, and cure rates of 98 % can be achieved if 3D histology is used [17, 18]. Note, pretreatment of the tumor with imatinib will cause tumor cell regression (but not to a tumor cell apoptosis); therefore, the peripheral tumor infiltration might not be detectable in 3D histology.

Merkel Cell Carcinoma, Adnex Tumors of the Skin (e.g., Microcystic Adnex Carcinoma), or Very Rare Soft Tissue Tumors

For these types of tumors, solid data of local treatments are missing, because these tumors are too rare. Interestingly, Merkel cell carcinoma seems to appear more frequently in the last years, and as a continuous infiltration of these tumors is assumed, 3D histology can be used to avoid local overtreatment. However, a primary safety margin width of 10 mm is recommended [19]. Immunostaining with CK 20 can be useful.

Table 8.3 summarizes the types of tumors which are suitable for 3D histology and which primary resection margins are reasonable. A rule of thumb in the treatment of all skin tumors should always be: The larger the tumor, the larger the safety margin has to be, and the more distinguished the location, the smaller width is useful in order to save important structures.

Stains for Different Tumor Entities

In addition to hematoxylin–eosin (H&E) staining, which is routinely used, some tumor types require special staining techniques for cryo-sections or paraffin-embedded material. It should be noted that due to the poorer quality, cryo-sections are generally more difficult to investigate without special staining methods (Table 8.4).

TABLE 8.3 Margin widths of special tumor entities depending on tumor size and location

1. Basal cell carcinoma >10 mm diameter	1–6 mm
2. Squamous cell carcinomas	1–10 mm
Desmoplastic type without or with perineural infiltration	4–10 mm
3. Recurrent tumors	3–10 mm
4. Lentigo maligna	1–6 mm
Lentigo maligna melanoma	2–6 mm
Acral lentiginous melanoma	2–6 mm
Desmoplastic melanoma	4–10 mm
5. Dermatofibrosarcoma protuberans	5–20 mm
6. Merkel cell carcinoma	5–20 mm
7. Extramammary Paget's disease	5–10 mm
Bowen disease perianal and genital	5–10 mm

TABLE 8.4 Special stainings

1. Basal cell carcinoma infiltrative types	Ber-EP 4
2. Squamous cell carcinomas with poor differentiation. Desmoplastic type or perineural infiltration	Cytokeratin 5/6, 5/14
3. Lentigo maligna, lentigo maligna melanoma, acral lentiginous melanoma, desmoplastic melanoma	Melan A
4. Dermatofibrosarcoma protuberans	CD 34
5. Merkel cell carcinoma	Cytokeratin 20
6. Extramammary Paget's disease	Cytokeratin 7

See also "e-immunohistology" in the Internet

Recurrent Tumors

Usually recurrent tumors have a more extended infiltration than primary tumors. But this infiltration is very often highly asymmetric and not predicable. Therefore, it is useful to perform first a "mapping" operation to determine the direction of the infiltration. The width of infiltration depends from the tumor type as well.

References

1. Keyvan N, editor. Mohs micrographic surgery. London: Springer; 2012.
2. Breuninger H, Dietz K. Prediction of subclinical tumour infiltration in basal cell carcinoma. J Dermatol Surg Oncol. 1991;17:574–8.
3. Breuninger H, Schaumburg-Lever G, Holzschuh J, Horny HP. Desmoplastic squamous cell carcinoma of skin and vermillion surface: a highly malignant subtype of skin cancer. Cancer. 1997;79: 915–9.
4. Häfner HM, Moehrle M, Eder S, Trilling B, Rocken M, Breuninger H. 3D-Histological evaluation of surgery in dermatofibrosarcoma protuberans and malignant fibrous histiocytoma: differences in growth patterns and outcome. Eur J Surg Oncol. 2008;34:680–6.
5. Lichte V, Breuninger H, Metzler G, Haefner HM, Moehrle M. Acral lentiginous melanoma: conventional histology vs. three dimensional histology. Br J Dermatol. 2009;160:591–9.
6. Boehringer A, Leiter U, Metzler G, Moehrle M, Garbe C, Breuninger H. Extramammary Paget's disease: extended subclinical growth detected using three-dimensional histology in routine paraffin procedure and course of the disease. Dermatol Surg. 2011;37:1–10.
7. Häfner HM, Breuninger H, Moehrle M, Trilling B, Krimmel M. 3D histology-guided surgery for basal cell carcinoma and squamous cell carcinoma: recurrence rates and clinical outcome. Int J Oral Maxillofac Surg. 2011;40:943–8.
8. Woerle B, Heckmann M, Konz B. Micrographic surgery of basal cell carcinomas of the head. Recent Results Cancer Res. 2002;160: 219–24.
9. Brantsch KD, Meisner C, Schönfisch B, Trilling B, Wehner-Caroli J, Röcken M, et al. Analysis of risk factors determining prognosis of cutaneous squamous-cell carcinoma: a prospective study. Lancet Oncol. 2008;9(8):713–20.
10. Leibovitch I, Huilgol SC, Selva D, Hill D, Richards S, Paver R. Cutaneous squamous cell carcinoma treated with Mohs micrographic surgery in Australia: I. Experience over 10 years. J Am Acad Dermatol. 2005;53:253–60.
11. Zollo JD, Zeitouni NC. The Roswell Parc Cancer Institute experience with extramammary Paget's disease. Br J Dermatol. 2000;42: 59–65.
12. Breuninger H, Schaumburg-Lever G, Schlagenhauff B, Stroebel W, Rassner G. Patterns of local horizontal spread of melanomas.

Consequences for surgery and histopathologic investigation. Am J Surg Pathol. 1999;23:1493–8.

13. Cohen LM, McCall MW, Zax RH. Mohs micrographic surgery for lentigo maligna melanoma. A follow-up study. J Dermatol Surg. 1998;24:673–7.

14. Moehrle M, Dietz K, Garbe C, Breuninger H. Conventional histology versus 3D-Histology in Lentigo maligna melanoma. Br J Dermatol. 2006;154:453–9.

15. Jahn V, Breuninger H, Garbe C, Moehrle M. Melanoma of the ear: prognostic factors and surgical strategies. Br J Dermatol. 2006;154: 310–8.

16. Jahn V, Breuninger H, Garbe C, Maassen MM, Moehrle M. Melanoma of the nose: prognostic factors, three-dimensional histology, and surgical strategies. Laryngoscope. 2006;116(7):1204–11.

17. Gloster HM, Harris KR, Roenigk RK. A comparison between Mohs micrographic surgery and wide surgical excision for the treatment of dermatofibrosarcoma protuberans. J Am Acad Dermatol. 1996;35: 82–7.

18. Hafner J, Schütz K, Morgenthaler W, Steiger E, Meyer V, Burg G. Micrographic surgery (Slow Mohs) in cutaneous sarcomas. Dermatology. 1999;198:37–43.

19. Boyer JD, Zitelli JA, Brodland DG, D'Angelo G. Local control of primary Merkel cell carcinoma: review of 45 cases treated with Mohs micrographic surgery with and without adjuvant radiation. J Am Acad Dermatol. 2002;47:885–92.

Chapter 9
Terminology and Facts

Definition of the Term "Microscopically Controlled Surgery"

Mohs termed the excision of tumor tissues with the aid of a histological evaluation "microscopically controlled surgery" (MCS), and in its original meaning it is different from the "ver tical serial cutting" (loaf-bread technique, see below). A horizontal serial cutting method was described by Burg and Konz in which the tumor would be cut horizontally using a microtome (see below). This has the advantage that the entire tumor can be analyzed histologically with only very small gaps.

Two-Dimensional Serial Techniques

Here the tumor specimen is cut in a series either of 1–3 mm wide vertical cuts using a scalpel (like cutting through a loaf of bread, hence also "loaf-bread technique") or horizontally with the microtome. Each of these sections is then embedded and analyzed histologically. If the tumor is sliced in very thin sections, i.e., 1 or 2 mm vertically (horizontal sections are tight together naturally), this technique may result in a sufficient sensitivity to detect all tumor outgrowths. However, the larger the excised tumor specimen is, the thicker will be the slices to

H. Breuninger, P. Adam, *3D Histology Evaluation of Dermatologic Surgery*, DOI 10.1007/978-1-4471-4438-0_9, © Springer-Verlag London 2013

avoid an exorbitant extra effort. These thicker slices introduce a much larger diagnostic gap and therefore are much more likely to be false negative. This is in strong contrast to the described 3D histology in this book where the entire tumor margin without any gaps will be evaluated. To keep track of the topographic orientation of each slice, all serial sections have to be well documented and marked with dye markers using special protocols like drawings for documentation and/or clearly defined rules of embedding. Documentation and communication with this technique can be done pretty similarly to the previously described procedures in 3D histology. Also here the communication using time logic for orientation or clear drawings are immensely helpful.

Serial Vertical Cutting, "Loaf-Bread Technique"

Also in this technique the removal of the tumor is done together with the safety margin. However, instead of isolating the margin and the tumor base separately for the histological evaluation, the excised specimen is divided into a series of parallel cuts, i.e., in strips of 2–4 mm width (Fig. 9.1a). These

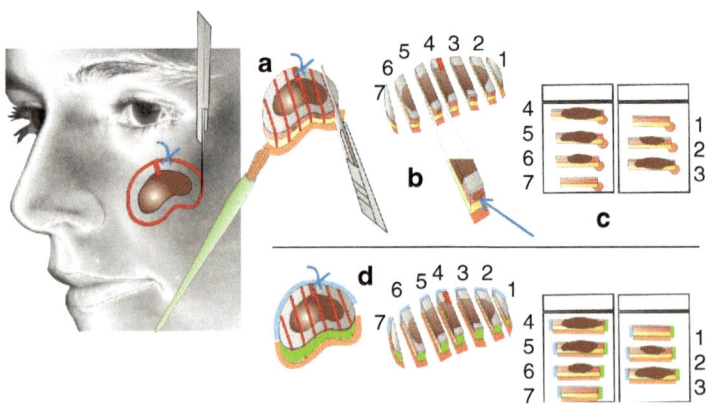

FIGURE 9.1 Serial vertical cutting, "loaf-bread technique", above using one side marking, below using complete dye marking

strips are then marked for orientation, divided for embedding, and histologically evaluated (Fig. 9.1b, c, or d with dye markings for orientation). In the example here none of the evaluated sections showed a tumor outgrowth at the margins of the analyzed strips. However, as indicated in Fig. 9.1b small tumor outgrows can be expected within one of the strips. Figure 9.1d shows the use of a complete dye marking of all excisional margins of the specimen.

However, a large number of sections are required to completely investigate the entire tumor. Therefore, the analysis of larger tumor specimens becomes quickly very labor intensive. Furthermore, the reconstitution of the original tumor and topographic orientation can be very challenging. Therefore, the effort which is needed for a serial section or "loaf-bread method" and the here described 3D histology is similar. In larger tumors 3D histology is even easier to do and will definitely provide a full histological evaluation.

Serial Vertical Cutting Versus 3D Histology (Comparison)

A direct comparison of the serial vertical cutting versus 3D histology highlights the similarities and differences between these techniques. The excision of the tumor in both techniques is identical (Fig. 9.2b). Only after the excision when the material is prepared for the histological evaluation the methods vary. The serial cutting requires in this example only two cassettes to fix the seven cuts in a fixed order for orientation which each of them have to be evaluated (Fig. 9.2a). 3D histology will require three cassettes as the base is fixed independently, but only five cuts have to be evaluated (Fig. 9.2b).

It is able to pick up the small indicated tumor outgrowth in the margin. In the vertical sectioning method, this outgrowth is missed as it is growing in the gap between two sections (blue arrow in Fig. 9.2a).

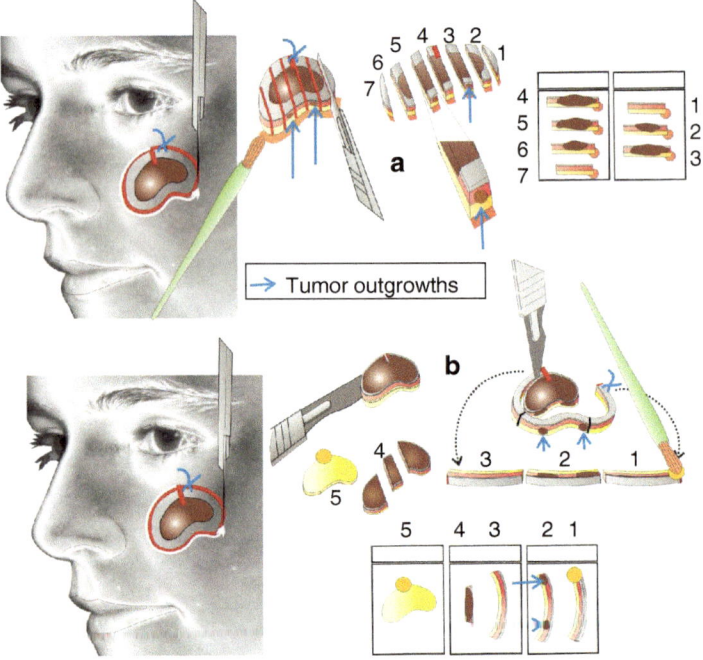

Tumor outgrowths

FIGURE 9.2 Serial vertical cutting versus 3D histology. The latter is easier to investigate

Serial Horizontal Cutting

In this method the tumor is first excised with one incision together with the safety margins at the side and base. First a small part of the center of the tumor is cut for diagnostics (Fig. 9.3a). The remaining two parts are then entirely embedded comparable to the embedding of the base in the 3D histology, i.e., with the base up for a cryo-sections or the other way round in paraffin embedded tissue (Fig. 9.3b). Now the entire tumor is sectioned from the base up to the epidermis and evaluated histologically for tumor outgrowths (Fig. 9.3c). Similarly to the 3D histology described here, this method enables the surgeon to analyze the entire margin of the excised tumor. Therefore, also here tumor outgrowths can be

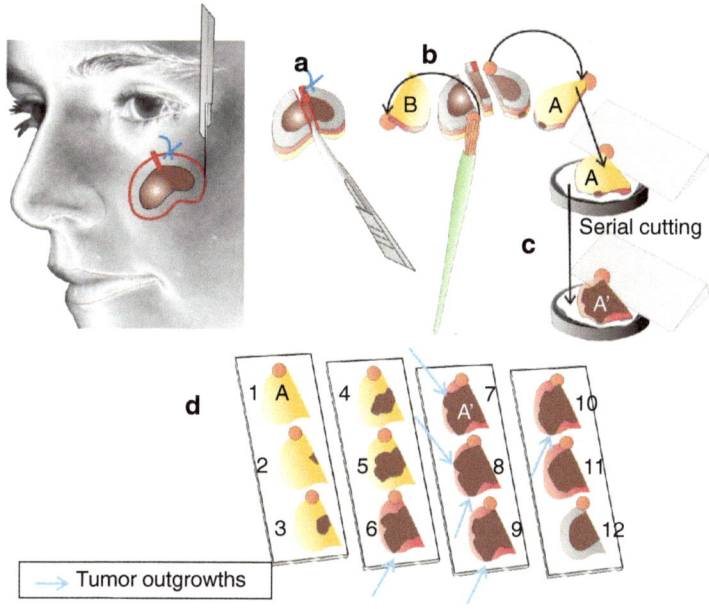

FIGURE 9.3 Horizontal serial cutting

detected fairly reliable (arrows in Fig. 9.3d). However, as the entire tumor has to be sectioned, many more sections have to be analyzed.

Final Remarks

Only methods which provide complete 3D histological evaluation of the entire margin of the excised tumor specimens can be truly termed "3D histology". Maybe the most profound difference between 3D histology and the vertical serial cutting technique is that the first is more likely to produce false-positive tumor margins, whereas the latter is more likely to produce false-negative tumor margins. However, so far a significant influence on tumor-free survival has not yet been confirmed by prospective, randomized clinical studies for larger tumors. For smaller tumors the difference was very low [1]. Nevertheless the success and significant higher healing rates in using the 3D histology are documented in an overwhelming amount of publications [2]. Also, the amount of time required for the 3D histological workup is not higher compared to other methods. Only a 3D imagination by the persons involved is necessary.

3D histology enables the full evaluation of the entire tumor margins without gaps. Therefore, it is highly recommendable for any malignant tumor, particularly if located at problematic locations or if the defect closure is likely to be difficult. 3D-histology methods are highly sensitive to detect tumor infiltrations, even very fine strands in very large tumors, and due to the relatively easy reconstitution of the margins in this technique very precise in predicting the localizations of such strands. Limitations exist if tumors infiltrate with single cell tumor strands which are histologically not detectable and if bone tissue is infiltrated. Here a histological evaluation is only possible after demineralization of the removed fragments.

The workflow of all methods shown can be divided between different departments. In general this is much more efficient and splits the required expertise. Here only clear rules for the handling of the tissue samples and the documentation have to be enforced. The documentation shown here using a simple clock logic for orientation has been proven itself as immensely powerful and works highly efficiently in our hands.

References

1. Smeets NWJ, Krekels GAM, Ostertag JU, Essers BAB, Dirksen CD, Niemann FHM, et al. Surgical excision vs Mohs micrographic surgery for basal-cell carcinoma of the face: randomized controlled trial. Lancet. 2004;364:1766–72.
2. Thissen MRTM, Neumann MHA, Schouten LJ. A systematic review of treatment modalities for primary basal cell carcinomas. Arch Dermatol. 1999;135:1177–83.

Index

H. Breuninger, P. Adam, *3D Histology Evaluation
of Dermatologic Surgery*, DOI 10.1007/978-1-4471-4438-0,
© Springer-Verlag London 2013

129